TECHNICAL REPORT

The Costs and Benefits of Moving to the ICD-10 Code Sets

MARTIN LIBICKI,
IRENE BRAHMAKULAM

TR-132-DHHS

March 2004

Prepared for the Department of Health and Human Services

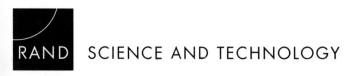

RAND SCIENCE AND TECHNOLOGY

The research described in this report was conducted by the Science and Technology Policy Institute (operated by RAND from 1992 to November 2003) for the Department of Health and Human Services, under contract ENG-9812731.

ISBN: 0-8330-3585-1

The RAND Corporation is a nonprofit research organization providing objective analysis and effective solutions that address the challenges facing the public and private sectors around the world. RAND's publications do not necessarily reflect the opinions of its research clients and sponsors.

RAND® is a registered trademark.

Published 2004 by the RAND Corporation
1700 Main Street, P.O. Box 2138, Santa Monica, CA 90407-2138
1200 South Hayes Street, Arlington, VA 22202-5050
201 North Craig Street, Suite 202, Pittsburgh, PA 15213-1516
RAND URL: http://www.rand.org/
To order RAND documents or to obtain additional information, contact
Distribution Services: Telephone: (310) 451-7002;
Fax: (310) 451-6915; Email: order@rand.org

Preface

In spring 2003, the National Committee on Vital and Health Statistics (NCVHS) asked the RAND Corporation to conduct a study of the benefits and costs of switching from ICD-9-CM (International Classification of Diseases, 9th Revision, Clinical Modification) codes for diagnoses and procedures to code sets based on the 10th revision of ICD: ICD-10-CM and ICD-10-PCS (International Classification of Diseases, 10th Revision, Procedure Classification System). This technical report presents RAND's first-order analysis of the benefits and costs of mandating such a switch (of both codes—either simultaneously or sequentially).

The primary audience for this report is the NCVHS and the community of those interested in health care informatics standards.

About the Science and Technology Policy Institute

Originally created by Congress in 1991 as the Critical Technologies Institute and renamed in 1998, the Science and Technology Policy Institute is a federally funded research and development center sponsored by the National Science Foundation. The S&TPI was managed by RAND from 1992 through November 2003.

The Institute's mission is to help improve public policy by conducting objective, independent research and analysis on policy issues that involve science and technology. To this end, the Institute

- Supports the Office of Science and Technology Policy and other Executive Branch agencies, offices, and councils
- Helps science and technology decisionmakers understand the likely consequences of their decisions and choose among alternative policies
- Helps improve understanding in both the public and private sectors of the ways in which science and technology can better serve national objectives.

In carrying out its mission, the Institute consults broadly with representatives from private industry, institutions of higher education, and other nonprofit institutions.

Inquiries regarding the work described in this report may be directed to the address below.

Stephen Rattien
Director, RAND Science and Technology
1200 South Hayes Street
Arlington, VA 22202-5050
Phone: (703) 413-1100 x5219
Website: www.rand.org/scitech/

The RAND Corporation Quality Assurance Process

Peer review is an integral part of all RAND research projects. Prior to publication, this document, as with all documents in the RAND technical report series, was subject to a quality assurance process to ensure that the research meets several standards, including the following: The problem is well formulated; the research approach is well designed and well executed; the data and assumptions are sound; the findings are useful and advance knowledge; the implications and recommendations follow logically from the findings and are explained thoroughly; the documentation is accurate, understandable, cogent, and temperate in tone; the research demonstrates understanding of related previous studies; and the research is relevant, objective, independent, and balanced. Peer review is conducted by research professionals who were not members of the project team.

RAND routinely reviews and refines its quality assurance process and also conducts periodic external and internal reviews of the quality of its body of work. For additional details regarding the RAND quality assurance process, visit http://www.rand.org/standards/.

Contents

Figures

Tables

Executive Summary

ICD-9 is the ninth revision of the International Classification of Diseases, a set of codes for recording the causes of mortality and morbidity. In the late 1970s, the United States developed a clinical modification of this code set (ICD-9-CM) and recently mandated its use for all diagnoses (Volumes 1 and 2 of ICD-9-CM). A third volume of ICD-9-CM was developed for procedures.

In 1993, ICD-10 was issued and it, too, was clinically modified to produce ICD-10-CM. A new standard, ICD-10-PCS (ICD-10, Procedure Classification System), was developed at the same time to succeed ICD-9-CM, Volume 3. Neither code set has yet been mandated for use. To help it advise whether such codes should be mandated, the National Committee on Vital and Health Statistics asked RAND the following questions:

- What are the costs and benefits of switching from ICD-9's diagnostic codes to those of ICD-10-CM?
- What are the costs and benefits of switching from ICD-9's procedure codes to those of ICD-10-PCS?
- If it is advisable to switch to both ICD-10-CM and ICD-10-PCS, should the switching be done sequentially or simultaneously?

Most observers believe that ICD-10-CM and ICD-10-PCS are technically superior to their ICD-9-CM counterparts. If nothing else, they represent the state of knowledge of the 1990s rather than of the 1970s. They have also been deemed more logically organized, and they are unquestionably more detailed—by a factor of two in diagnoses (and twenty for injuries) and by a factor of fifty in procedures.

Estimation of Costs

Change, even change to a superior code, is not free. Costs can be classified into three categories:

- costs of training
- productivity losses
- system changes.

We estimated the cost of training by identifying relevant groups—hospital coders, other coders, physicians, and code users. We then estimated how many of them would need to be trained and how long it would take to train people in each category. We made additional estimates for the initial and long-term loss of productivity among coders and physicians. We estimated the cost of systems reprogramming by sampling payers, providers, and software vendors; dividing their answers by membership (in the case of payers) or revenue (in the case of providers and software vendors); and extrapolating to the entire population. Table S.1 represents our estimate of the one-time and cumulative annual costs of switching to ICD-10-CM and ICD-10-PCS. Note that annual costs are not discounted over time.

The third column in Table S.1 represents the additional costs required to change first to ICD-10-CM and then to ICD-10-PCS; these additional costs come largely from the need to complete testing and systems integration twice rather than once. We see no offsetting benefits from switching sequentially.

Thus, our best guess is that the cost of conversion will run $425 million to $1,150 million in one-time costs plus somewhere between $5 million and $40 million a year in lost productivity.

Table S.1
Summary of Estimated One-Time Costs and Cumulative Annual Costs[a]

	Personnel	Cost Estimate ($ million)	Additional Cost of Sequential Change ($ million)
Training	Full-time coders	100–150	0–20
	Part-time coders	50–150	
	Code users	25–50	0–10
	Physicians	25–100	
Productivity losses	Coders	0–150[a]	
	Physicians	50–250[a]	
System changes	Providers	50–200	5–50
	Software vendors	50–125	5–20
	Payers	100–250	5–50
	CMS[b]	25–125	5–20

[a] Cumulative total of ten years of annual costs (undiscounted).

[b] CMS = Centers for Medicare and Medicaid Services.

Estimation of Benefits

To develop benefit estimates, we developed a set of parameters based on plausible—but by no means inevitable—scenarios, to account for five major classes of benefits:

- More-accurate payments for new procedures
- Fewer miscoded, rejected, and improper reimbursement claims
- Better understanding of the value of new procedures
- Improved disease management
- Better understanding of health care outcomes (considered, but not estimated).

These benefits were calculated over a ten-year period (the historic time between successive versions of ICD).

Such benefits largely come from the additional detail that ICD-10-CM and ICD-10-PCS offer. However, to realize those benefits, providers must use the full codes, use them correctly, and use them in a fashion that is neutral to the reimbursement system. ICD-9-CM is by no means always completely, correctly, or neutrally exploited.

More-accurate payments for new procedures could be a benefit for the following reasons: New procedures cannot get a code in ICD-9-CM (which is running out of room); they are more expensive than the procedures they would replace; and they are therefore not fully reimbursed and not always performed for Medicare/Medicaid patients (and for those covered by payers using similar payment standards)—even though they are cost-effective. For this scenario, we estimated the benefits total at $100–1,200 million.

The case for fewer erroneous, rejected, and exaggerated claims is based on the tendency for ICD-10-CM, and particularly ICD-10-PCS, to be less ambiguous and more logically organized and detailed than their predecessors. However, erroneous, rejected, and questionable claims are likely to rise in the initial confusion; it may take five years to see positive cumulative benefits. For this scenario, we estimated the benefits at $200–2,500 million for fewer rejected claims and $100–1,000 million for fewer exaggerated claims.

ICD-10-PCS could help in understanding the value of new procedures that will no longer be lumped in with old procedures, as they often were in ICD-9-CM. The assumption is that analyzing hospital discharge records would permit providers and payers to determine how effective such procedures are and for which populations. This would shift when and where they are performed (e.g., ineffective procedures would be done less often; effective ones would be extended to new patients) with net benefits as a result. For this scenario, we estimated the benefits total at $100–1,500 million.

By permitting more-detailed billing records, ICD-10-CM would help payers and providers more easily identify patients in need of disease management and more effectively tailor disease management programs. Our disease management scenario focused on diabetes, both for its prevalence and for the sixfold expansion in the number of diabetes codes available in ICD-10-CM. Roughly 60 percent of the benefits came from putting more of the right people in such programs, and the rest came from refining disease management for those already in a program. Assuming that diabetes accounts for two-thirds of the total disease management benefits (there was far less expansion of codes for heart disease, for instance), we put the benefits total at $200–1,500 million.

We considered other potential benefits—such as the help that better codes give to research on health care, improvements in the ability to rate providers, and an enhanced ability to detect emerging diseases—but could assign no reasonably plausible benefit to them.

Table S.2 on the next page summarizes our benefit calculations.

Conclusions

It is likely that switching to both ICD-10-CM and ICD-10-PCS has the potential to generate more benefits than costs. But the estimates for costs—and, in particular, the parameters for benefits—are subject to considerable variation.

Table S.2
Summary of Estimated Benefits over a Ten-Year Period[a]

Category	Benefit ($ million)	Largely Due to
More-accurate payment for new procedures	100–1,200	ICD-10-PCS
Fewer rejected claims	200–2,500	both
Fewer fraudulent claims	100–1,000	both
Better understanding of new procedures	100–1,500	ICD-10-PCS
Improved disease management	200–1,500	ICD-10-CM`

[a] Benefits are not discounted over time.

Acknowledgments

Thanks are due to the many people who took the time to explain thc vagaries of code sets to us and detailed the impact that changing them might have on their operations. Special thanks are due to our project sponsors at CDC, Donna Pickett and Marjorie Greenberg, without whose expert knowledge and deep memory banks we would have made far less progress on this work. Further thanks are due to our reviewers, George Goldberg and Lee Hilborne. Finally, the work could not have been done without the enthusiasm, counsel, and patience of Helga Rippen, who headed S&TPI during the period this report was written.

Acronyms and Abbreviations

AAHP	American Association of Health Plans
AHA	American Hospital Association
AHIMA	American Health Information Management Association
AHRQ	U.S. Agency for Healthcare Research and Quality
APC	Ambulatory payment classification
AR-DRG	Australian Refined Diagnosis Related Group
CCI	Canadian Classification of Health Interventions
CCP	Canadian Classification of Procedures
CDAC	clinical data abstracting center
CDC	Centers for Disease Control and Prevention
CIHI	Canadian Institute of Health Information
CMG	case-mix group
CMS	Centers for Medicare and Medicaid Services
CPT	Current Procedure Terminology
DRG	diagnosis related group
ETG	episode treatment group
FAH	Federation of American Hospitals
FI	fiscal intermediary
GAO	General Accounting Office
HbA1c	Hemoglobin A1c
HCFA	Health Care Financing Administration
HCUP	Healthcare Cost and Utilization Project
HEDIS	Health Plan Employer Data and Information Set
HFMA	Healthcare Financial Management Association
HHS	Department of Health and Human Services

HIC	health identification claim
HIPAA	Health Insurance Portability and Accountability Act of 1996
HMO	health maintenance organization
ICD-9	International Classification of Diseases, 9th Revision
ICD-9-CM	International Classification of Diseases, 9th Revision, Clinical Modification
ICD-10	International Classification of Diseases, 10th Revision
ICD-10-AM	International Classification of Diseases, 10th Revision, Australian Modification
ICD-10-CA	International Classification of Diseases, 10th Revision, Canadian Modification
ICD-10-CM	International Classification of Diseases, 10th Revision, Clinical Modification
ICD-10-PCS	International Classification of Diseases, 10th Revision, Procedure Classification System
ICDO-3	International Classification of Diseases for Oncology, Third Edition
IT	information technology
LMRP	local medical review policy
MEDPAR	Medicare Provider Analysis and Review
NCHS	National Center for Health Statistics
NCVHS	National Committee on Vital and Health Statistics
NEC	not elsewhere classified
NOS	not otherwise specified
PPO	preferred provider organization
VA	Veterans' Administration
WEDI	Workgroup for Electronic Data Interchange
WHO	World Health Organization
XML	Extensible Markup Language
Y2K	year 2000

CHAPTER ONE

Introduction

In 2001, medical care in the United States consumed $1.4 trillion dollars, employed roughly 12 million people directly, and generated petabytes of information. All this care must be paid for, and what the nation is getting for its health care dollars should somehow be assessed. . This assessment requires that the complexities of health care be reduced to a set of diagnostic and procedure codes. In three to six alphanumeric characters, those codes must bear the burden of description for this complex system.

Two code sets dominate today's official documentation of health care interventions.[1] One is ICD-9-CM (ICD stands for the International Classification of Diseases). Volumes 1 and 2 of this code set deal with diagnoses. Volume 3 covers procedures with a focus on inpatient procedures.[2] The other code set is the CPT® (Current Procedure Terminology), which describes outpatient procedures and inpatient services reported directly by physicians. The CPT is owned by the American Medical Association.

The first two volumes of ICD-9-CM are clinical modifications (CM) of the international standard, ICD-9, which itself was developed in 1977 by the World Health Organization (WHO) to record mortality statistics (it is the 9th revision of a standard that is now a century old). It has been in use in the United States since 1979. The standards of both ICD-9-CM and the CPT are based on the state of knowledge in the mid-1970s, and it is fair to note that medical knowledge has advanced considerably in the past 30 years. Because of continuing advances, ICD-9-CM cannot help but fall increasingly behind the present state of knowledge, despite annual updates. Diagnoses are incorrectly organized, and their implied etiology is often incorrect (e.g., many diseases are now known to be of mitochondrial origin). New procedures (for instance, certain laparoscopies) are not uniquely identified; instead, they are classified within the same code developed for older procedures (e.g., open surgeries) and thus are not easy to pick out or analyze separately.

ICD-9-CM, Volume 3, in particular, has the reputation of lumping together a large number of different procedures. For example, Nelly Leon-Chisen of the American Hospital Association testified before the National Committee on Vital Health and Statistics (NCVHS) on April 9, 2002, that "Code 99.29[3] . . . is used to report a variety of procedures

---

[1] Separate specialized code sets are used in specific medical fields, such as psychology and dentistry. Inputs for materials such as supplies and devices are accounted for using other coding systems, e.g., the health care procedure coding system (HCPCS). We do not examine other coding systems in this report.

[2] Under Health Insurance Portability and Accountability Act (HIPAA) regulations, Volume 3 is required only for facility or institutional reporting of inpatient procedures. However, it also covers outpatient procedures.

[3] Code 99.29 is "injection or infusion of other therapeutic or prophylactic substance."

such as an injection of epinephrine to cauterize a rectal ulcer, infusion of a narcotic into a pump for pain relief, insertion of an implant in the eye for slow release of an antiviral drug, and injection into the uterine artery to treat a fibroid." Echoing that observation, Sue Prophet-Bowman of the American Health Information Management Association (AHIMA) added that Code 81.47 (other repairs of the knee) included "both open and arthroscopic repairs. Numerous types of aneurysm repairs are classified in Code 39.52. . . . All types of destruction of skin lesions including that by [excision], laser, cryosurgery, cauterization, and fulguration are classified to 86.3, other local excision or destruction of lesion or tissue of skin and subcutaneous tissue."

In addition, new devices go unseen by the system. Until a drastic change was made in a 2002 revision, there was no way to encode the implantation of a cardiac pacemaker/defibrillator except by recording the implantation of both devices as if there had been two separate surgeries.

In 1992, WHO issued a new version of its mortality code, ICD-10. Seven years later, ICD-10 became the official U.S. standard for recording mortality data. Between 1994 and 1996, clinical modifications were made to that standard, creating ICD-10-CM for classifying diagnoses. At the same time, the Centers for Medicare and Medicaid Services (CMS) decided to revamp the entire system of classifying inpatient procedures and developed what it called ICD-10-PCS. As a consequence, the structures of both ICD-10-CM and ICD-10-PCS are based on scientific knowledge that was current in the early to mid-1990s rather than in the late 1970s.

The Health Insurance Portability and Accountability Act of 1996 (HIPAA) gave the Department of Health and Human Services (HHS) the responsibility for designating a standard code set with which to describe diagnoses and procedures. At the time, ICD-10 was not deemed mature enough to be mandated,[4] and so ICD-9-CM was chosen instead. This choice in no way was meant to prejudice the eventual move to ICD-10. Nevertheless, the transition to ICD-10-CM and ICD-10-PCS did not take place as soon as its proponents would have liked. Thus, the issue remains under advisement by the NCVHS.

Study Objective

In support of NCVHS's decisionmaking process, this report addresses the following questions:

- What are the costs and benefits of switching from ICD-9's diagnostic codes to those of ICD-10-CM?
- What are the costs and benefits of switching from ICD-9's procedure codes to those of ICD-10-PCS?
- If it is advisable to switch to both ICD-10-CM and ICD-10-PCS, should the switching be done sequentially or simultaneously?

---

[4] Various features add maturity to a code: The code has been widely reviewed and commented on; it has been experimented with and shown to be consistent; it has been through "beta-testing," and one can teach and learn it.

To answer these questions, RAND was asked to assess the implications of implementing ICD-10-CM and ICD-10-PCS for current ICD-9-CM users, including the costs and benefits of the change (both quantifiable and nonquantifiable). The task consisted of

- identifying affected entities and the degree to which they would be affected
- identifying costs, including opportunity costs, associated with the transition—including, but not limited to, information system changes, rate negotiation, recalculation of reimbursement methodologies, training, and changes to forms
- considering the timing of transition, including the impact of timing options on costs and benefits, potential return on investment, and interaction with other major health information investment tasks
- identifying immediate and future costs and benefits of improved data for—but not limited to—patient safety, outcomes analysis, reimbursement, disease management, utilization review, and health statistics
- contacting affected entities including the National Center for Health Statistics (NCHS), CMS, and other third-party payers, to acquire their assessments of costs and benefits within their own organizations.

It is important to be clear about what this report does *not* address. First, it deals with actual rather than notional coding systems. Our primary job is not to go back and redesign ICD-10-CM or ICD-10-PCS or even to study what features they should or should not have. We had to deal with the choices that were presented to us. That said, one of the arguments for not making the switch today is the possibility that it would be more cost-effective to write a new equivalent of ICD-10-CM and/or ICD-10-PCS and implement it a few years later than to implement the current version of ICD-10-CM and/or ICD-10-PCS now.

Second, the report deals only with the switch between ICD-9 and ICD-10—not a switch between ICD-10 and any other coding system (e.g., CPT). In other words, we are asking *not* whether ICD-10 is the best coding system to switch to but only whether, based on a tally of costs and benefits, switching is worthwhile at all.

Third, and correspondingly, we do not deal with any transition between coding standards other than ICD-9 and ICD-10. We assume that if another coding standard is used now—e.g., CPT—the same standard will be used afterward (even though shifts may well be made). Outpatient procedures not already coded in ICD-9 will, we assume, not be coded in ICD-10.

What Is Counted in a Cost-Benefit Analysis?

We must also be explicit about what a cost-benefit analysis includes. Ideally, after all the calculations of costs and benefits are made and the estimates completed, a ratio of benefits to costs is arrived at based on economic criteria—for instance, a figure of 1.47 would indicate that the switch is worthwhile; alternatively, 0.78 would indicate that the costs outweigh the benefits. For reasons that will become clear below, we cannot honestly report such precise numbers. Some categories of costs and benefits (e.g., the cost of training) can be estimated with some degree of confidence; other costs and benefits are difficult to estimate, and the estimates are not entirely meaningful (e.g., the effect of new codes on the quality of studies that measure health outcomes).

A key assumption of a cost-benefit analysis is that the analysis is being considered from the perspective of the public in general, not from that of any one sector. For instance, changes in transfer payments unaccompanied by changes in the cost of providing services are irrelevant to a cost-benefit analysis. By a similar accounting logic, correcting (or, alternatively, exacerbating) misalignments between the cost of performing a service and the reimbursement for such a service is—*up to a point*—neither a cost nor a benefit. Someone gains and someone loses. But beyond some point, misalignment between the cost of providing a service and how much money providers are allowed to collect for it *is* a cost. Large, frequent, or systematic misalignments could lead to "deadweight losses"[5]—the distortions that occur when people adjust their behavior to artificial prices rather than to the true cost of providing a service.

Finally, if reductions in fraud can be credited to a shift to new codes, they count as a clear benefit (and vice versa). There is a general moral consensus that fraud should not be considered a transfer payment that merely washes out in the calculations: Payers lose; the gains to fraudulent providers do not count; and the ethical tone of the profession suffers.

Some of the arguments against ICD-10 (specifically, ICD-10-PCS) hold that a switch would result in complex and costly renegotiations between payers and providers over the cost of various services. Renegotiations may not be necessary if the new codes can be mapped into the old codes precisely. Yet the transition may create the opportunity for one side or the other to bring up the issue. If the other side is not in a position to refuse outright and if raising the issue involves true negotiation costs (everything else being transfer payments), it is not clear that such costs should be counted on the negative side of the cost-benefit ledger.

To summarize, the following are *likely* to count as costs:

- additional requirements for training
- additional work effort
- large, frequent, and systematic differences between prices and costs.

In contrast, the following are *unlikely* to count as costs or benefits):

- changes in transfer payments (unaccompanied by changes in effort or resources)
- work effort (e.g., renegotiations) prompted by, but not required by, a change in codes
- small, infrequent, or random differences between prices and costs.

---

[5] In economic terms, deadweight loss is the net loss in social welfare that results when goods and services are used whose value does not justify the costs of producing them or are forgone despite the fact that their value exceeds the cost of producing them.

Methodology

Our primary methodology had three steps:

1. Identify the major categories of both costs and benefits
2. Estimate the amount of money involved in cost category
3. Characterize and develop a scenario for each benefit category.

We relied on three basic data sources for our work:

- We built on testimony before the Subcommittee on Standards and Security of the National Committee on Vital and Health Statistics (including written submissions), notably but not exclusively on April 9–10, May 29–30, June 26, and August 28–29, 2002.
- We conducted 80 interviews with a total of 90 people between the beginning of April and the beginning of August 2003 (see Appendix B). This group included experts plus a sampling of affected parties (e.g., association representatives, providers, payers, software and service vendors, and government officials).
- We conducted a literature search with the primary goal of determining how and how well ICD-9 codes were used. The results, indicated in the Bibliography, point to several general themes. One set of readings indicated how researchers used ICD codes in determining broad parameters and trends in public health. Another set specifically evaluated the accuracy and relevance of ICD-9 codes (primarily but not exclusively diagnostic codes) and pointed out many problems in their use.

Estimation of Costs

The methodologies we used for estimating costs and benefits were consistent with one another but not identical. As more fully explained below, most of the costs are either for training or for changing systems. We estimated training costs by determining how many people would need training and for how long; we multiplied this figure by the cost of employing trainers (plus travel and expenses where appropriate). We estimated systems costs by polling a representative sample of payers, providers, and software vendors and generating a ratio of expected costs to operator size (number of members for payers; revenues for providers and software vendors). This method produced more consistent results for payers than for providers and software vendors.

Estimation of Benefits

Our methodology for developing a scenario of benefits varied for each major category shown in Table S.2 and is described separately in each section of Chapter Three. Broadly speaking, we started with the universe—(e.g., the number of procedures done, the cost of administering health insurance, the number of diabetic patients, etc.) and multiplied it by several percentages. Prominent among those percentages is a parameter that represents the percentage of cases likely to be affected by specific attributes associated with the switch between ICD-9 and ICD-10. In many cases, these percentages are unknown or unknowable in advance of a switch. We therefore offer these parameters to (1) indicate an order-of-magnitude effect, and (2) indicate where further research may be useful.

Organization of the Report

We begin with the analysis of costs in Chapter Two. Chapter Three presents a number of benefits of a transition to ICD-10 and the breadth of those benefits. Chapter Four compares the rationale for making a switch to both coding sets simultaneously with making them sequentially. Chapter Five presents our conclusions, and Chapter Six notes some transition strategies.

Several appendices have also been supplied to aid the narrative. Appendix A contains background material in three areas: how codes are used, how ICD-10-CM and ICD-10-PCS differ from their predecessors, and some issues involved in mapping from one code to another. Appendix B contains the list of interviewees.

CHAPTER TWO

Estimation of Costs

This chapter considers several categories of putative costs:

- training
- lost productivity among coders
- systems changes.

Each of these categories, in turn, can be divided into subcategories. Among the people who would require training, for instance, are professional coders employed in hospitals, the larger but less-involved population of those who work for clinics and physicians' offices entering diagnostic codes, and code users at payer organizations.

There has been considerable testimony that the costs of switching to ICD-10-CM and ICD-10-PCS would be extensive in the sense that many activities would be affected by the switch. Jim Daley from Blue Cross/Blue Shield of South Carolina provided NCVHS with a long list of areas that might be affected: payer software (screens, databases, reports, queries, adjudication, reimbursement, data groupers, statistics, reference); provider software (for scheduling, billing, claims submission, finance, intensive care unit/emergency room activity, decision support); reimbursement determinations (diagnosis related groups [DRGs]—see Appendix A for discussion, APCs [ambulatory payment classifications], line-pricing by procedure, contract negotiations, determinations of medical necessity, disease management policies, actuarial research); training (claims processors, administrative staff, medical review staff, actuaries, auditors, fraud investigators, physicians, nurses, coders, laboratories, employee benefits administrators); and statistics (trend analysis, utilization management, rating, quality-of-care, HEDIS [Health Plan Employer Data and Information Set], and provider profiling).[1] Nevertheless, *extensive* does not necessarily mean *expensive* if the cost of any one activity is relatively small (e.g., only a few people are involved).

We chose to aggregate rather than to make individual estimates of each separate small-cost category on the grounds that even a robust individual estimate would in many cases be dwarfed by the estimation errors in the larger categories.

---

[1] "ICD-10 Impacts to the Health Care and Insurance Industry," presentation to the NCVHS meeting of August 29, 2002.

Requirement for Additional Training

Although few coders could begin to use ICD-10 with full efficiency right away, the amount of training that coders will need will depend on the settings in which they work. The amount of training required for coders has been well studied, and results from other countries can serve as benchmarks, as discussed below.

Full-Time Coders

We begin with ICD-10-PCS, an inpatient—and thus, for the most part a hospital-related—standard. To generate a proxy number of full-time coders, we used the 50,000 coders currently employed by hospitals, on the theory that few outpatient facilities have enough volume to keep coders employed full-time.

The time to get full-time coders to proficiency in both new codes has been estimated, by AHIMA and others, at several days to a week. If such retraining costs $2,500—split between expenses ($500) and lost work-time ($2000)[2]—the cost is roughly $125 million[3]—50,000 × $2,500. Incidentally, most of today's coders have been expecting clinical versions of ICD-10 to be mandated ever since ICD-10 itself was promulgated. So, most coders have long expected the transition.

No empirical data exist concerning which standard can be taught more quickly to *new* coders. Advocates of ICD-10-PCS say that its logical structure makes it easier to learn. Nevertheless, it does have more content because there are more individual codes from which to choose. In either case, the actual codes constitute only a small amount of what coders need to learn, and turnover in the profession is low, perhaps less than 10 percent a year.[4]

Confidence Range: We believe a confidence range of ± 25% is appropriate. On the one hand, some hospital coders may not receive formal training. On the other hand, some people who receive formal training may be from other parts of the health care industry: teachers, consultants, and selected coders from outpatient facilities. So we estimate the range as $100 million to $150 million.

Part-Time Coders

Calculations for what training is required for people to code only ICD-10-CM are somewhat less exact. Such coders work in outpatient settings and in home health-care agencies. The roughly 200,000 doctors' offices translate to roughly 200,000 coders. Yet because most outpatient settings are specialized in some way, it is rare for an office to deal with more than a few hundred diagnostic codes. Some even have preprinted or at least preformatted forms

---

[2] Statistics from AHIMA (www.ahima.org/members_only/member_profile_data.cfm) suggest that the average income of coders is $45,000 a year or $25 per hour over 1800 hours. Using a standard ratio of 2 to 1 for fully burdened employment costs yields a cost of $50 per hour or $2,000 for a 40-hour week.

[3] Gail Graham of the Veterans' Administration, reporting on tests of ICD-10-PCS with coders, observed that good coders had no problems with the switch but that this was not so when coders had deficient knowledge of anatomy and physiology. Bolstering those coders' knowledge of such fundamental subjects would take several months, with a cost closer to $10,000 each or higher. Multiplying the least proficient 20 percent of coders (10,000) by the cost of intensive training would yield another $100 million or thereabouts. That said, there is no evidence that such training was required in Canada, where a similar but somewhat smaller transition was made in coding procedures.

[4] Chris Frazier of the American Association of Procedural Coders observed to the NCVHS (May 29, 2002): "At our national conference this year . . . most [coders] predominantly were over five years, some 10, 15 years. It seems that people . . . stay in the profession once they do have the certification."

("superbills") on which the correct diagnosis is checked off. In many cases, physicians' offices do not record diagnoses with a high degree of specificity. It is not uncommon for physicians presented with a choice of 40 different diabetes codes (in ICD-9-CM) to use the most general code in creating billing statements, even though more-specific codes convey more information. For such offices, little or no training will be required because only a few codes are ever used.

Because ICD-10-CM (compared with ICD-10-PCS) is less of a departure from ICD-9-CM, AHIMA has estimated the retraining time for people for whom coding is an ancillary duty at four to eight hours.[5] Some will simply train themselves as they go; using the Web as the instructional vehicle may also make potential efficiencies in training available. Multiplying 200,000 coders by the sum of a $100 training cost and $400 in lost productivity (8 hours × $50/hour) yields $100 million.

Confidence Range: The two sources of variation are the percentage of part-time coders to be trained (we assumed one person per doctor's office) and the number of hours that each would need. The figure of $100 million represents the high end of the four-to-eight-hour range, but requirements for two to four days' worth of training for ICD-10 coders were also advanced in the aforementioned AHIMA/AHA study. So we report a range of $50 million to $150 million.

Training Code Users and Physicians

Code users may also need some time to become familiar with the new codes. The largest single group of users consists of the employees of payer organizations, whose ranks can be estimated at roughly 250,000, perhaps just 150,000 of whom work directly with codes. It is unclear how much training they will get; many were never trained in ICD-9-CM. To some extent, employers may count on the tendency of people to associate codes and descriptions over time (e.g., as seen together on printed forms or in computer systems) to help familiarize them with their equivalents in ICD-10. In any case, no payer has mentioned contemplating a formal training program (although, to be fair, since no ICD-10 requirement has yet been levied, and most payers are thinking instead about the impending need to meet HIPAA requirements). If the average employee needs the same amount of training that ICD-10-CM coders would get (i.e., four to eight hours), the number of person-years consumed in training could be approximated at 600 (again, using the eight-hour figure), at a cost of $50 million.

Concerning the retraining of physicians, one observer felt that, at the high end, each physician would need four hours of education on the new diagnostic codes plus two further two-hour sessions in the first year, for a total of eight hours. Another responder indicated that the requirement for training would depend on how different ICD-10-CM was from ICD-9-CM. If multiplied by the half-million physicians in clinical practice, this sums to

---

[5] To be precise, our estimate was not for an ICD-10-CM coder as such but for those who only code part-time, a description that characterizes the vast majority of those who code for the 200,000 physicians' offices (with the possible exception of very large clinics that perform no inpatient procedures but that have enough outpatient procedures to keep a coder employed full time). In summer 2003, AHA and AHIMA together studied ICD-10-CM coding and polled the coders, almost all of whom were full-time coders (or coding teachers and consultants) on how much training they believed was needed. On average, the coders wanted 2-1/2 days of training (wanting something, of course, is not the same as successfully getting others to pay for it). This is an almost entirely different group from the part-time coders in physicians' offices—most of whom deal with only a fraction of the codes handled by hospital coders, teachers, and consultants. Thus, the full-time coders' desired time of 2-1/2 days is not inconsistent with the eight-hour estimate we use to calculate costs.

roughly 2,000 person-years of training at a cost of $500 million.[6] It is more likely that only a few doctors would want training to familiarize themselves with how to comply with new code requirements. A plausible estimate is that training would be requested by only one in ten doctors—notably, physicians who deal with injuries (where there is a large expansion in diagnostic codes) and surgeons (because more information is needed on complex procedures to satisfy ICD-10-PCS). None of the physicians we talked to said that they themselves would have to be retrained. In fact, professional coders are extremely leery of doctors doing their own coding.[7] Finally, as noted, many physicians' offices, for better or worse, rely on super-bills to record their diagnoses. We therefore used a figure of $50 million for this category.

Confidence Range: The greatest source of uncertainty concerns, primarily, the percentage of code users and physicians who would be trained and, secondarily, the time they would need for training. The $50 million estimate for code users assumed 100 percent participation and eight hours training—both figures probably on the high side. The $50 million estimate for physicians, however, assumed only 10 percent participation and thus has potential for a wide confidence range. So, we report $50 million to $150 million as the range for coders and physicians combined.

Impact on Productivity

Coder Productivity

The new coding systems, notably ICD-10-PCS, have been widely praised as a more logical system than their predecessors and, thus, are presumably easier to work with. To the extent that this is true, people will be more productive. Nevertheless, because ICD-10-PCS asks for more bits of information per code (and thus more this-or-that choices to be made) and offers more codes from which to choose, there is reason to believe that the process of working from computer-based menus will take longer *even after* people have become used to ICD-10-PCS.

CMS formally tested ICD-10-PCS in 1998 by using two clinical data-abstracting centers (CDACs): DynKePRO of York, PA, and FMAS Corporation of Columbia, MD. In the first round, 2,500 records were coded by each CDAC to generate feedback to 3M Health Information Systems (the company that developed ICD-10-PCS). In the second round, 100 records were coded in both ways to compare ICD-9-CM to ICD-10-PCS in terms of time to code and other criteria (e.g., number of codes required, how much information each produced, general strengths and weaknesses). DynKePRO's report indicated that no "significant time difference in coding was found between ICD-9-CM and ICD-10-PCS." FMAS, however, found that ICD-10-PCS generated more codes[8] than did ICD-9-CM (2.48 per patient vs. 2.16 per patient) and that each record, on average, took longer to code (3.6 minutes versus 1.9 minutes). This 1.7-minute difference, however, is only an initial point on the learn-

---

[6] Since most physicians are required to take a minimum number of hours of continuing medical education, some may elect to count this training against what they would have had to do anyway. But the training is still not free because it displaces other training that presumably has some value.

[7] This suggests that ICD-10-PCS, which is almost always coded by full-time professionals, is less pertinent to the issue of physician training than ICD-10-CM would be.

[8] In contrast, many of the new codes in ICD-10-CM are substitutes for having to put down two or more codes in ICD-9-CM to describe a condition such as diabetes.

ing curve. There is no good way to know how quickly coders will move down the curve as they get more experience.

Multiplying the FMAS numbers—which suggest that coders will spend 1.7 more minutes of coding per patient, at least initially—by the 1.8 million discharges a month that have procedures associated with them[9] suggests that 50,000 extra coder hours will be required the first month that ICD-10-PCS is in effect. At a fully burdened cost of $50 an hour per coder,[10] this translates into $2.5 million in additional costs the first month. Assuming a six-month learning curve, over which 60 percent of the difference disappears, the break-in costs (the difference between productivity loss in the first few months and long-term productivity losses) would be roughly $5 million, and the additional long-term costs from reduced productivity would be $10 million a year.

The growing use of automated encoders may reduce the loss of productivity from the code switch. These encoders use a branching-tree logic. A coder enters clinical terms to describe a condition (e.g., neoplasm, pancreas). The computer then offers the coder a menu to refine the choice (which, in turn, may result in more choices). When the menus are completed, the computer selects a code and enters it into the record. QuadraMed, a leading supplier of such software, has nearly a thousand hospitals as customers, which it believes make up 20 percent of the market. After accounting both for differences in defining the market and for the tendency of larger hospitals to be more automated, the conclusion remains that more coding takes place with computer assistance than without it.

As of this writing, there has been no comparable testing of ICD-10-CM, although AHIMA and AHA were in the process of conducting a test over the summer of 2003. However, both Canada and Australia provide some real-world examples, as noted below.

Confidence Range: The precision of these calculations must be qualified by the observation that 200 records is a very small sample upon which to base conclusions (especially when the other study showed no difference). Although a six-month learning curve is consistent with practice in Canada and Australia (see below), the premise that one-third of the productivity loss is more-or-less permanent has less backing. So we report $0 to $15 million as the range of annual productivity loss for coding.

Canada and Australia as Benchmarks for Coder Productivity Cost Estimates

Like the United States, Canada has new diagnosis and procedure codes. Canada's counterpart to ICD-10-CM, ICD-10-CA, consists of ICD-10 plus 6,000 codes. This number is similar to—but somewhat smaller than—the number added in the United States to make ICD-10-CM (as tallied in the 1997 crosswalk), indicating that changes in diagnoses are comparable. Canada's counterpart to ICD-10-PCS, CCI (Canadian Classification of Health Interventions) is a less ambitious expansion. Although CCI is built on a conceptual foundation similar to that of ICD-10-PCS—hierarchical construction of primitives and classification largely by body part—it has only 17,000 codes, compared with the 120,000 codes of

---

[9] National Center for Health Statistics, *Ambulatory and Inpatient Procedures in the United States 1996,* November 1998, p. 4. For other good statistics see www.cms.hhs.gov/reports/hcimu/hcimu_07142003.pdf (see also the 2001 National Hospital Discharge Survey: www.cdc.gov/nchs/about/major/hdasd/nhds.htm). Comparable statistics are also available from the State of California's Office of Statewide Health Planning and Development (see www.oshpd.cahwnet.gov/HQAD/HIRC/patient/discharges/index.htm).

[10] Where coders are in short supply, the extra hours may come out of overtime rather than regular salary, and thus this figure could be somewhat higher.

the U.S. ICD-10-PCS. Still, CCI represents a sixfold expansion over its predecessor, the Canadian Classification of Procedures (CCP). A further difference is that coding in Canada is used for statistical purposes rather than for billing. Canada's single-payer policy also means that coders spend far less time than U.S. coders operating under guidelines that indicate which diagnoses and procedures a patient's insurer will process easily and which they will balk at. However, as noted, Canada *does* have a DRG-like case-mix group (CMG) system for financing hospitals (Ontario, for instance, is beginning to use case-mix statistics to measure the relative productivity of its hospitals with a view toward rewarding the more productive ones).

As of mid-2003, Canada was more than halfway through its transition to ICD-10 (every province came on board separately; Manitoba and Quebec have yet to switch). In preparation for the switchover, Canadian coders were given preparatory material, a two-day workshop, post-workshop material, a one-day refresher course, and options for special workshops and teleconferences. There was an initial loss of productivity, but it disappeared after several months. The province of Ontario trained 1,100 coders. The coding environment is fairly uniform across Canada. All coding is electronic, but the level of automation is equivalent to using an electronic book (e.g., akin to Adobe Acrobat's ".pdf" file.) Indeed, there was one electronic book that the government (Canadian Institute for Health Information [CIHI]) passed out to everyone. The Canadian experience was that coders became sufficiently proficient with the new codes well inside six months, with no reported loss in long-term productivity. As such, estimates that each U.S. coder would need a week's worth of training are not inconsistent with Canada's experience of three days plus extras.

Australia's experience is similar, although the change Australian coders went through was fairly modest: from 12,500 to 14,000 disease codes and from 3,600 to 6,000 procedural codes. As with Canada, introduction was staged, with the more densely populated states in the southern part of the country switching in 1998 and the rest in 1999.

Physician Productivity: Potentially Greater Work Required for Some

Coding itself is inherently a process of translating from words to symbols, capturing the essence but not retaining the details. The patient record has far more detail in it than is reflected by the codes. Most of the detail in it is irrelevant to the characterization of the patients' diagnoses and even procedures. Coding necessarily compresses information; in doing so, information is lost.

ICD-10, both for diagnoses (ICD-10-CM) but especially for procedures (ICD-10-PCS), is designed to capture more information than ICD-9 does. It makes finer distinctions and loses less information that was present in the patient record. However, the benefit of losing less information comes with the possibility that coding may require physicians or nurses to add information to the patient record (one respondent talked in terms of "more physician input into the coding process"). If the information is broadly useful, then there are offsetting gains in having it recorded. But if the information is only useful to the extent needed to satisfy an imposed standard (i.e., physicians otherwise would not record such information), it counts as a cost. This requirement for more information is less likely to affect the recording of diagnostic information in ICD-10-CM, which retains most of the not otherwise specified (NOS) and not elsewhere classified (NEC) codes of its predecessor, and is more likely to characterize ICD-10-PCS, which has drastically reduced such unspecified codes.

The cost of mandating additional information on patients' records is hard to estimate. If ICD-10 comes into use, there is bound to be greater dialogue between coders and caregivers on how to classify specific diagnoses and procedures. In some cases, notably for procedures, coders will ask for more information. So, both coders and physicians would have to do more work (at least until both get used to what information is required to code correctly). Nevertheless, even though this process seems harder on coders—who have to ask the questions and wait until they get the answers—there have been no complaints from that community, which suggests that the amount of extra information required, even during the break-in period, is unlikely to be great. To generate cost figures for extra physician work we assumed that, at the beginning: (1) 80 percent of all patient records have only routine procedures or have sufficiently documented ones, (2) coders faced with inadequate patient records will contact physicians half of the time, and (3) five minutes of physician time is necessary to resolve matters. We multiplied the estimates based on these assumptions by the nation's aforementioned 1.8 million monthly hospital discharges, leaving an additional 20,000 physician-hours a month. If the combined cost for physicians and coders is $200 an hour, this entails $4 million worth of extra work. Over time, physicians will learn what additional information to add in such cases without having to be asked. Based on the same assumption that only a third of the additional work persists after six months, this number declines to an estimated $16 million a year.

Confidence Range: The estimate has sources of imprecision: the percentage of discharges that need additional physician input to be coded, the amount of time (i.e., the five minutes) required to resolve the average discharge, and the earlier assumption that a third of the added work is permanent. So we report $5 million to $25 million per year as the range.

System Changes

System Changes for Providers

Hospitals and clinics, among others, will have to alter their billing and administrative systems to handle new codes, which are longer and contain alphanumeric characters. Most providers, however, buy their systems from vendors, and most of the provider-vendor relationships have a software maintenance component. Thus, most providers look to their vendors to update their systems on a periodic basis. Many providers, however, would bear additional expenses for planning, end-user services (e.g., report generation), testing, ensuring backward compatibility with earlier data, and systems integration.

As a general rule, the level of concern over the impending costs to switch to ICD-10 has been modest, with many providers saying, in effect, that their vendors would take care of it. In testimony, neither the American Hospital Association (AHA) nor the Federation of American Hospitals (FAH) raised serious cost concerns over systems changes (they were more concerned with training costs). Major hospital chains were relatively unconcerned about the change, believing that they would need little additional consulting—if any—and that their major cost would be testing and integration. One hospital chain (representing 0.5 percent of the total U.S. inpatient market) estimated the cost of testing and integration at a maximum of one person-year. Another said that it would be "close to a trivial event." The Veterans' Administration (VA), which accounts for roughly 3 percent of the total potential patient population in the United States, does not anticipate that accommodating the switch from ICD-9-CM to ICD-10-CM/ICD-10-PCS will cost it more than $1 million (thanks in part to the fact that the VA's computer systems have been recently revamped). But there were also outliers among hospitals (e.g., "easily a million dollars worth of work"). A $100-million transition cost may well be plausible (even when including costs borne by providers with in-house systems).

Confidence Range: For most hospitals, the cost of a systems changeover will run roughly $1 per annual discharge. But to the extent that outliers account for a disproportionate share of the costs, estimates would be difficult to generate on the basis of small sample sizes. We therefore must use a broad range of $50 million to $200 million to accommodate such an effect.

The Cost of Software Changes

A large share of the cost of adapting provider systems will fall to system and software vendors, who will ultimately pass that cost along to their clients. The transfer may, however, be hard to trace even in retrospect. Many software vendors that provide maintenance contracts will update their software for no additional charge to respond to government mandates. Nevertheless, Bob Hardesty (Cerner) testified before the NCVHS (May 29, 2002) that

> In general, we do not charge additional software license fees for the design, development, or software modifications related to government regulatory change. This is covered under our ongoing agreements for maintenance support and is believed to be a fairly common approach among the vendor community. However, given the broad impact of the change of this nature, it would be expected that there would be professional service fees involved for activities undertaken involving planning, testing, training, conversion, and implementation.

A rough estimate of the cost of adaptation, extracted from information taken from two major vendors, suggests that from design to final testing would take three years and would involve, over the course of that period, up to 10 percent of the software labor force, engaged in this software project perhaps an average of one year over the entire three-year period. A third major vendor has cited a rough estimate of 50 to 100 person-years for total adaptation to ICD-10. Other vendors, however (e.g., QuadraMed, Cerner, Solucient, CorSolutions, Symmetry, and Ingenix), suggest that this may overstate the cost of adaptation. They talk in terms of a few person-years of effort, even among those suppliers with major market shares.

Under the circumstances, we estimate the total cost of adapting software to bring providers from ICD-9 to ICD-10 at no more than $100 million.

Confidence Range: The two sources of inaccuracy stem from the limited sampling base and the necessarily imprecise estimates offered. In addition, these estimates come from specialists in health informatics and not the larger systems integrators (e.g., IBM, Siemens, EDS). Nevertheless, outcomes are more likely to be lower than higher. So, we use $50 million to $125 million as the range.

System Changes for Payers

Although changing payer systems may well constitute the single largest category of costs for a switch to ICD-10, estimates of the costs are by no means clear. Many payers, all of whom realize that ICD-10 is coming, are nevertheless unsure of what the change means. They are even unsure of whether it represents a change in field size and composition, are unfamiliar with the existence of crosswalks between old and new code, and do not know whether or not the new code set is a 1:N expansion. Many payers are still struggling with accommodating the impact of HIPAA on their systems, an experience that has made them somewhat sensitive to what seem to be the large but uncounted costs of dealing with new codes.

Overall, payers represent a widely varied group. Some, generally the larger ones, develop and maintain their own systems; others rely on vendors. As a general rule, such transitions cost more among those who develop their own systems, especially those that have invested considerable time and money in mainframe computer systems and have thereby achieved efficiency at the expense of flexibility. The twin burdens of accommodating Y2K and HIPAA persuaded many payers to upgrade their overall systems—many in favor of vendor products[11]—rather than continue to patch what they had. But many legacy systems remain. Two respondents are actively seeking new computer systems that can be built to accommodate ICD-10 without conversion; in neither case, however, was ICD-10 capability specifically asked for.

New codes carry two types of costs: (1) costs for accommodating a code set, characterized by a larger field size and alphanumeric characters and (2) costs for reprogramming the logic that previously used ICD-9-CM codes.[12] Hard as it may be to believe for those used to quickly changing field sizes in popular microcomputer programs, it is not straightforward to make such changes in mainframe programs and to ensure that all the variables manipulate the data correctly. One payer representative estimated that merely expanding field size by a character accounted for two-thirds of the overall costs of adopting an updated code. The other third of the cost is for replacing the logic by which procedures are considered covered based on their accompanying diagnoses. This cost arises not only in programmer time, but in the time required to make new eligibility decisions in those cases where one-to-many-N mappings do not apply.[13]

Our estimate was based on conversations with eight payers, representing a mix of health maintenance organizations (HMOs) and preferred provider organizations (PPOs). The following is offered with the caveat that the costs of switching over to ICD-10 have yet to be calculated by many payers (even those who have asked that the government first estimate the total costs to the economy of such a switch before mandating it). That noted, these numbers have a certain consistency.

The eight payers we talked to fell into three groups. The first (three respondents with collectively 4 percent of the market) are counting on their software vendors to make the changes for them. The second (three respondents[14] with collectively 12 percent of the mar-

---

[11] Many respondents, including software vendors, supported this contention.

[12] There may also be costs entailed in running both old and new codes through payer systems at the same time. Nevertheless, if there is one changeover date, this should be a short interval after the new codes are in effect for new discharges, during which claims for old cases are being settled.

[13] Where one-to-many mappings do apply, the N relevant codes can always be substituted by the one prior code as a short-term response. There will also be cases where the additional detail of ICD-10-CM and/or ICD-10-PCS will permit payers to make finer differentiations and therefore refine the eligibility rules—even where one-to-many expansion prevails. One must presume, however, that payers see sufficient benefit in such a change and therefore accrue no net cost in making it.

[14] One company generated two estimates, one of 40 cents per member and the other of 80 cents per member. The higher estimate is indirect. Although the respondent suggested that it would cost "hundreds of millions of dollars" to rebuild the

ket) need to invest roughly 40 cents per client member. The third (two respondents with collectively 3 percent[15] of the market) need to invest roughly $1 per member. Based on the three groups combined, the costs of adapting software to accommodate ICD-10 would run $150 million if extrapolated to the entire payer base.[16]

It should be noted that at least one section of the insurance business, the fiscal intermediaries (FIs) that handle claims for CMS, has *already* been required to accommodate code lengths as long as seven digits in anticipation of ICD-10-PCS. Thus, their expenditures are sunk costs and are not counted toward the prospective costs of the decision to switch from ICD-9 to ICD-10.

A contrast with experience in Canada and Australia may prove illustrative. Ontario's cost of switching from ICD-9 to ICD-10-CA was originally estimated (circa 1995) at $5 million Canadian (roughly $3–4 million U.S.). At that price, switching was deemed unaffordable if paid for directly by the provincial government. Reexamination of the policy suggested, however, that the costs may have been overstated and could be borne by hospitals without affecting the rates paid for health care in the province. Extrapolating from that set of (perhaps inflated) numbers to the U.S. population (and ignoring the many differences between the Canadian and U.S. health care systems) yields a figure of roughly $100 million as the total systems cost for the switch. Australia reports having spent roughly $3 million Australian ($2 million U.S.) to switch to the new diagnostic and procedure codes, a sum comparable to $30 million U.S. in population-adjusted figures.[17]

Confidence Range: Eight payers is a small sample size under the circumstances, and the HIPAA experience (in which costs outran estimates) has prompted many respondents to err on the side of overestimation. Nevertheless, the consistency in the numbers led us to use $100 million to $250 million as the appropriate range.

System Changes for CMS

As of late July 2003, CMS had yet to determine how it was going to accommodate the switch to ICD-10 or what that switch would cost (it was anticipated that cost estimates would be provided department by department by CMS). A good deal depended on how CMS proposed to use crosswalks, at least in the period prior to what are expected to be major revisions of the DRGs based on ICD-10.

CMS does not administer patient care reimbursement directly; it relies on FIs to handle the paperwork and on various carriers to process physician claims. The FIs are regional, and there are subtle but complex differences in what combination of diagnoses and procedures they cover. Local medical review policies (LMRPs)—local adjustments to na-

---

company's logic action, this estimate had yet to consider many possible options such as using a crosswalk from the new to the old for reducing the cost. The 80-cent figure was generated by extrapolating from the two to three full-time-equivalent employees required to keep up with annual updates of ICD-9 plus CPT (ICD-9-CM, Volume 3, plays a minor role in the company's logic)—and estimating that the switch from ICD-9-CM to ICD-10-CM was equivalent to 20 to 30 years' worth of updates.

[15] One of the two respondents was sized based not on its total membership alone but also on the membership of those organizations for which it processed claims.

[16] Since State Medicaid agencies can be considered tantamount to payers, and since their "membership" was subsumed in the calculations above, the transition costs should be included in the above estimate—if their per capita costs are in line with those of private payers.

[17] These data do not include the cost borne by the several dozen private insurers in Australia, but private insurers play a much smaller role in Australia than their U.S. counterparts do.

tional (i.e., CMS) standards in the area of what constitutes medical necessity—are mostly based on ICD-9-CM codes. If those codes change, the logic of the LMRPs must also change. Where the crosswalk to the new code is straightforward, the change is trivial. For others, more work may be required. There are roughly 100 total contractors (FIs and carriers combined), each with multiple separate policies. Changing all those policies will have a cost. Nevertheless, periodic contract renegotiations are the norm in this industry, with one-year and three-year cycles being quite common. Thus, although the conversion to ICD-10 is more likely to introduce more things to negotiate over, it is far less likely to spur negotiations when there otherwise would have been none.

Confidence Range: At this time, we can only guess at the cost to CMS. In effect, it is a placeholder until CMS makes its own estimate. We therefore have to use a very broad estimate of $25 million to $125 million for CMS.

Summary of Costs

Table 2.1 summarizes the major cost categories and the expected cost ranges for each.

We estimate that the one-time cost of a switch will run $425–1,150 million. The loss in productivity on the part of hospital coders and physicians could run $5–40 million a year once the initial six-month break-in period ends. (In Chapter Four, we present a separate estimate for the additional cost of switching from ICD-9-CM to ICD-10-CM and ICD-10-PCS sequentially rather than simultaneously.)

Issues have been raised over how evenly costs would be distributed. As a rule, we found that the likely costs of accommodating a code change are roughly proportional to the number of patients the providers see or the number of members that payers have. The most significant source of unevenness we found is from owners of systems the size and age of which make them relatively difficult to change (irrespective of how efficient they are at their

Table 2.1
Summary of Estimated One-Time Costs and Cumulative Annual Costs[a]

	Personnel	Cost Estimate ($ million)	Additional Cost of Sequential Change ($ million)
Training	Full-time coders	100–150	0–20
	Part-time coders	50–150	
	Code users	25–50	0–10
	Physicians	25–100	
Productivity losses	Coders	0–150[a]	
	Physicians	50–250[a]	
System changes	Providers	50–200	5–50
	Software vendors	50–125	5–20
	Payers	100–250	5–50
	CMS	25–125	5–20

[a] Cumulative total of ten years of annual costs (undiscounted).

current tasks). In general, however, these firms are well-established and thus in the best position to shoulder the costs.

We also were not able to detect or predict any systematic shift in payments as a result of the change in coding between ICD-9 and ICD-10. Current plans suggest that Medicare DRGs will not be redefined until some time after ICD-10 goes into effect. CMS pays for 47 percent of all hospital costs (2002 data), which militates against any large immediate shift in reimbursement rates.

CHAPTER THREE

Estimation of Benefits

When asked to state the benefits to Australia of moving to ICD-10-AM, Dr. Rosemary Roberts, director of the National Centre for Classification in Health at the University of Sydney, listed the following:[1]

- Currency. ICD-9-CM is based on ICD-9, a WHO classification published in 1978. ICD-10 itself is now ten years old (it was published in 1992). So much of the terminology and structure of ICD-9 and ICD-9-CM is out of date. Although ICD-9-CM is maintained by NCHS and CMS, the basic framework is outdated and not always amenable to "fiddling at the edges." This has led to ICD-9-CM being regarded as a "for billing" classification rather than a clinical classification.
- International comparability with ICD-10 morbidity data
- National and international comparability with ICD-10 mortality data[2]
- Clinical credibility of the classification, in that the Australian clinical modification of ICD-10 (ICD-10-AM) results from a wide consultation with specialist clinicians and coders
- Better ability to describe new diseases and new understanding of diseases such as HIV, neoplasms, diabetes, injuries and external causes, drugs
- Ability to construct an Australian version of case-mix grouping (AR-DRG) based on current clinical knowledge and a mature and maintained classification
- Acceptance by clinicians and administrators of the AR-DRG composition (in code) and cost weights
- Expertise in clinical classification and terminology that will help us in the transition to use of clinical terminologies in electronic health records
- Development of standards for application of the classification that relate to current clinical practice
- Parity between terms used in health records and terms in the classification itself
- Use of classification in national morbidity data for research. The Australian Institute of Health and Welfare publishes annually "Australian Hospital Statistics," which

---

[1] E-mail from Rosemary Roberts, May 29, 2003.

[2] Despite the obvious benefits of having directly comparable mortality and morbidity statistics, differences in codes are not the only source of discrepancy. In the state of New York, for instance, doctors are constrained in what they can put on death certificates. If, say, the doctor knows that a patient died of sepsis but the test for the bacteria has not yet come back from the laboratory, no such cause can be listed, but nothing prevents the doctor from putting this diagnosis in discharge forms. That said, corrections can be submitted for death records after tests or autopsy results are received.

allows monitoring of disease patterns and utilization of health services. Specific research projects on prevalence of adverse events in hospital episodes, cause of death and general practice are one example of cross-setting use of ICD-10 and ICD-10-AM data. ICD-10-AM also includes the neoplasm updates from ICDO-3 [ICD for Oncology, Third Edition] so that recent knowledge on behavior of neoplasms is consistent with its classification in ICD-10. The same applies in mental health and the maintenance of ICD-10 with other WHO Mental Health publications.

Notwithstanding the correctness of such claims, none of them is particularly easy to associate with improvements in health or savings in cost, and they are much less easy to quantify—no small consideration when the cost of change can be measured in the hundreds of millions of dollars.

As a general rule, better information confers benefits only when it informs better decisions. Technically speaking, quantifying the benefits of better information requires, first, understanding which decisions are affected by such information, how they would have been made in the absence of such information, and how they are made with the new information; and second, determining the benefits resulting from the altered decisions. This process entails a great many levels of steps in a logic chain, variations in which frustrate measuring benefits exactly. Nevertheless, better decisions may still be worthwhile.

The next five sections discuss benefits in each of the following five categories:

1. More-accurate payments for new procedures
2. Fewer miscoded, rejected, and improper reimbursement claims
3. Better understanding of the value of new procedures
4. Improved disease management
5. Better understanding of health care outcomes.

For four of the categories (all except number 5), we created scenarios for the benefits that could conceivably be expected from CM and ICD-10-PCS. The numbers from the scenarios are estimated over the ten years following the adoption of the codes—ten years being the historic time between successive versions of ICD. As for category number 5, we concluded that, although there was a real benefit, there was no scenario that permitted numbers to be assigned to it.

We also examined two other putative benefits: (1) the improved ability to rate providers and (2) the ability to counteract emerging diseases and bioterrorism earlier, but we concluded that the new codes were unlikely to offer much help in those areas, for reasons we explain below.

In making and testing claims about benefits, it is important to be explicit about which factors in the new codes are the bases of the benefits. For instance, although improvements in the scientific categorization of diagnoses are all to the good, the real benefits, if they exist, would come from the greater (and/or more meaningful) specificity of the codes, which permits more patient information to be recorded and transferred.

More-Accurate Payments for New Procedures

As one researcher[3] has argued, "The predictive power and clinical utility of a DRG classification system is limited or empowered to a large extent by the precision of the available diagnosis and procedure codes." This dictum applies with particular force to the transition to ICD-10-PCS. If many more separate procedures can be coded, one could differentiate simple and complex inpatient procedures now lumped together. This differentiation introduces the possibility of paying for different procedures differently. In theory, this is a net plus, if procedures that would have been optimal for patient care were not performed because providers feared they would lose money by offering them.

CMS (which, as noted, funded 47 percent of all hospital expenses in 2002) is acutely aware that the exhaustion of ICD-9-CM, Volume 3, limits its ability to code innovative procedures uniquely. Many new techniques are far more complex and, hence, more expensive than are other procedures in the same DRG. In recent years, CMS has started a program to reimburse selected new procedures at rates higher than what is indicated by the DRGs such procedures are associated with. The limitations on expanding ICD-9-CM, Volume 3, are one major reason that very few such procedures have been approved (the fact that many are not very cost-effective or have not gotten FDA approval are other reasons). If and when ICD-10-PCS is approved, the number of procedures for which new codes are likely to be granted may rise to several dozen a year.

That noted, none of our respondents has indicated that they do not perform specific procedures because those procedures have been classified into the wrong reimbursement categories. It has also been pointed out that physicians bill using the more ample CPT rather than the code-constrained ICD-9-CM, Volume 3. To the extent that physicians, rather than hospitals, decide on what constitutes an appropriate standard of care, the impact of having sufficient ICD-10-PCS codes would be vitiated. Overall, it is fair to say that health care does not entirely conform to the economic models prevalent in other industries—given that 85 percent of all hospitals are nonprofit institutions.

A Benefits Scenario

To generate a scenario of benefits, it is necessary to know for each type of prospective procedure:

M = number of times the procedure would have been performed over the next ten years for patients covered by CMS if reimbursement was not an issue

P_{coded} = odds that such a procedure would merit one of the few new codes issued for procedures

$P_{notdone}$ = percentage of procedures not done because hospitals choose not to bear the financial disincentives of doing so (likely to be correlated with the difference between the cost and the reimbursement for such procedures)

B = net opportunity cost (measured in dollars) of not doing such a procedure

---

[3] See Muldoon, 1999.

The actual benefit is the product, over all new potential procedures, of: $(1 - P_{coded}) \times P_{notdone} \times M \times B$. In practice, this calculation requires estimating some number, M, as the number of performed procedures that are (1) unlikely to get their own codes, (2) have a net benefit, but (3) present cost challenges for hospitals—and then multiplying it by some balking percentage to calculate the number of procedures not done. This number is then multiplied by B, the net benefit per procedure, as averaged over this set.

To estimate M, we start with the CMS estimate that several dozen such procedures are likely to get new codes every year and then compare this to today's 3,500 procedure codes to get an idea of the percentage of procedures that would, in fact, have new codes. One must also take into account that although many codes encompass different procedures, innovators are unlikely to push for new codes if the new procedures are variations of old procedures and can generally be accommodated in ICD-9-CM, Volume 3. In other words, both the several dozen and the 3,500 are smaller parts of what may be larger numbers. One must also take into account the recent tendency for a large percentage of new procedures to be less invasive and thus, in the long run, less totally expensive than their predecessors. They are also more likely to be undertaken in ambulatory surgery centers, once physicians become familiar with performing them. So, in this scenario, we assume that 1 percent of all procedures in any given year are truly new (i.e., several dozen divided by 3,500 codes). Multiplying by 20,000,000 annual inpatient procedures yields 200,000 procedures introduced in any one year that are significantly different enough to merit their own codes in ICD-10-PCS. Counting only those covered by CMS—one-half—leaves 100,000 procedures. So M = 100,000.

Of the several dozen "new" procedures, we assume that three of them are of such high volume that they get their own codes. If the distribution, by count of procedures, follows Zipf's law,[4] then we further assume that these three account for 40 percent of the total number of procedures—that is, $P_{coded} = 0.4$. Removing this 40 percent (that is, multiplying by $1 - P_{coded}$) leaves 60,000 procedures.

As noted, the odds that a hospital would refuse to carry out an expensive but otherwise useful procedure are unlikely to be high, given that most hospitals are nonprofit and are used to averaging costs. Furthermore, many new procedures—at least after a few years of having been performed—may have costs comparable to or lower than their alternatives, and thus hospitals would have little reason not to perform them. Conversely, it is not unknown for providers to balk at taking Medicare and Medicaid patients because of cost issues. So, for the sake of argument we will use a figure of 10 percent as $P_{notdone}$. This leaves 6,000 procedures.

The next step is to estimate the benefits forgone from not doing such procedures. Assuming that every procedure performed has a net benefit and that the distribution of these benefits is exponentially distributed, most procedures are marginally beneficial whereas a few are hugely beneficial. It is also plausible that hospitals are more likely to carry out hugely

---

[4] Zipf's law suggests that certain statistics (e.g., the population of a nation's cities), when ranked from greatest (e.g., the population of metropolitan New York City) to smallest, have the following property: The sum of the first N of such statistics is proportional to the binary logarithm of N + 1. Thus, the population of the greatest number (e.g., the population of metropolitan New York City) is comparable to the sum of the next two (e.g., for metropolitan Chicago plus metropolitan Los Angeles) as well as the sum of the next four (e.g., for San Francisco, Philadelphia, Dallas, and Washington) etc. Thus, if the law is applied to our case, the most popular three procedures combined would be undertaken roughly 40 percent as often as the most popular 31 procedures.

beneficial procedures on which they lose money and balk at carrying out marginally beneficial procedures on which they lose money. So, again, for the sake of argument, we will estimate that the average procedure not done would have had a cost-benefit ratio of 1.5. At, say, $10,000 a procedure, this equates to a $5,000 net benefit. Multiplying everything together, the opportunity cost of not doing procedures for CMS patients during the first year because the procedures could not be coded would be $30 million.

This number, however, grows annually as more procedures are nominated for new codes and new codes accommodate only some of them. If 6,000 procedures are not done in the first year, 12,000 procedures will not be done the next year (i.e., two years' worth of nominated procedures), and 18,000 will not be done the year after that, etc. This suggests that the $30 million should be multiplied by 50 to generate an annualized ten-year benefit. But a 50-fold increase may be too high. Over time, new procedures may come down in cost (e.g., because of learning-curve effects) or low-cost variants may be developed for certain markets. So, a lower figure of 25-fold may be more appropriate for calculating a ten-year benefit. This produces a figure—with all due caveats—of $750 million.

Confidence Range. This estimate is subject to many forms of imprecision, such as the number of procedures performed that are truly new but do not merit their own codes, the value of performing such procedures, and the assumption that, in some cases, the costs of such procedures will decline to where hospitals are not losing money performing them. Nevertheless, the largest assumption is the 10 percent balking figure: it could be somewhat higher and could be a great deal lower as well. We therefore use a wide range of $100 million to $1,200 million to represent this benefit.

Fewer Miscoded, Rejected, and Improper Reimbursement Claims

Insofar as ICD-10-CM represents an incremental change whereas ICD-10-PCS is more radical, observable reductions in error rates, claim rejections, and fraudulent claims are more likely to occur in the reporting of the latter.

Fewer Miscoded Claims

Coding error rates are the difference between the reported code and the actual (correct) code for one or more diagnoses or procedures. ICD-10-PCS is at the least more logical than its predecessor; its hierarchical structure is more transparent. On the other hand, its coding structure will be new, and there are far more codes from which to choose. The General Accounting Office (GAO)[5] has argued that, by creating more categories—for the sake of argument, assume it is by adding a lowest-order digit—more errors will result. Yet, if these errors result from miscoding only on the nth digit, as long as one is aware of the possibility of error, one still gets more information from having an nth digit that is usually correct than from having no nth digit at all. The best guess at this point is that error rates are likely to *rise*

---

[5] From GAO, *HIPPA Standards: Dual Code Sets Are Acceptable for Reporting Medical Procedures*, GAO-02-796: "With more codes available for use, there are more opportunities for coding errors with inaccurate codes used in describing the procedures provided, particularly if the descriptions of procedures on medical records do not capture all the dimensions of the procedure needed to complete a code."

initially until people are familiar with the codes.[6] The improved logic and standardized definitions of ICD-10-PCS, the more accurate clinical terms in ICD-10-CM, and the more specific code descriptions of both all give reason to believe that error rates will eventually drop below where they are under ICD-9-CM—but exactly when that will happen is hard to predict.

The cost of reducing random error is difficult to quantify without knowing the consequence of such errors. If errors that are not caught result in erroneous payments and such uncaught errors are randomly distributed (people are as likely to overbill as to underbill), the effects are neutralized—nonrandom errors not large enough to bias the provision of medical care mean that the payers' gain will be the providers' loss and vice versa. If errors are caught, the result is likely to be a returned claim.

Fewer Returned Claims

Another potential benefit from switching from ICD-9 to ICD-10 is that fewer claims would be rejected and sent back for more information. By one estimate, only one in every five hospital claims is paid completely with no additional questions asked. As a report of the Workgroup for Electronic Data Interchange (WEDI) observed of ICD-9 in "Issues Surrounding the Proposed Implementation of ICD-10":

> There are increasing requirements for submission of documentation to support claims due to lack of sufficiently detailed information contained in code assignments; inability to collect data on new conditions or use of new technology due to insufficient space in ICD-9-CM for new codes; lack of quality data to support performance measurement, outcomes analysis, research, and all of the other uses of coded data (including particularly poor data regarding ambulatory and managed care encounters); increased opportunity due to the number of different conditions of procedures categorized to the same code (for example, an investigational procedure assigned to the same code as a non-investigational procedure); inability to effectively monitor service and resource utilization, analyze healthcare costs, monitor outcomes, and detect fraud—all of these things have costs associated with them. (p. 4)

> ICD-10-CM and ICD-10-PCS incorporate much greater specificity and clinical detail, which will result in significant improvements in the quality of the data used. This greater detail may help reduce the number of cases where copies of the medical record need to be submitted for clarification for claims adjudication. (p. 9)

Nevertheless, it is the consensus of almost everyone who commented on the matter that rejection rates are bound to rise initially as people unfamiliar with the codes enter the wrong code[7] and payers, who also have to learn new codes, err and reject correct codes.[8] At some point, the reduced rejection rate from more and better information will exceed the

---

[6] Some coders (particularly those with less training) who would otherwise question poor suggestions made by automatic encoders may be more inclined to accept them in ICD-10 until they get comfortable with the new codes.

[7] There are many ways to detect questionable coding, not least of which is a lack of correspondence between diagnoses and procedures or among primary and secondary diagnoses. Certain diagnoses can also be considered unexpected based on a patient's history.

[8] If people cannot recognize the difference between an ICD-9 and ICD-10 code—unlikely but not impossible—then some claims resubmitted by providers may be initially presumed to be two separate claims.

increased rejection rate from residual errors.[9] The crossover point could vary from six months to three years.

A Benefits Scenario

Reducing rejection rates is a benefit because it reduces the amount of work for payers and providers. To reiterate, the assumptions used for the calculations are that (1) a large percentage of the cost of processing reimbursements comes from the work required to adjudicate them, (2) the cost of a claim's adjudication is proportional to the number of cycles it makes (every claim makes at least one cycle from provider to payer), and (3) the switch to ICD-10, once its break-in period is over, can reduce the number of cycles the average claim makes. We further assume that better information can reduce the claims process by one cycle, at most. Hence the variables to be considered are

CSB =   reduction in the percentage of claims sent back

C =   average number of cycles a claim makes

CA =   overall cost of claims adjudication in dollars.

The actual benefits would be calculated as $CSB \times (CA/C)$, where CA/C is the average cost per cycle of processing a claim. CA is some large fraction of the total cost of health care financing (but it also includes providers' billing services). This equation assumes that each of N cycles costs the same to process as the first cycle does—in the face of arguments by some that follow-on cycles are less expensive (they only cover particular aspects of the claim, not the whole claim) and by others that they are more expensive (they are more likely to entail personal involvement rather than the operations of automatic systems.

We estimate CA at roughly $20 billion nationwide, bearing in mind that (1) only a fraction of the cost of administering insurance is in claims adjudication, but that (2) payers also have expenses for claims adjudication. If the average claim goes through two cycles, CA/C is $10 billion. Since we can only guess at the reduction in the send-back rate, it is therefore useful for understanding the potential rather than predicted benefits of better information.

So, for the sake of argument, we select a send-back reduction rate of 1 percent (e.g., if 45 percent of all claims were sent back under ICD-9, then only 44 percent are sent back once ICD-10-CM and ICD-10-PCS are in place). This yields an annual benefit of $100 million (1 percent × $10 billion).

As noted, however, the reverse is more likely to be true initially: more claims are likely to be sent back until people get used to ICD-10. So, multiplying $100 million by ten years to come up with a $1 billion total benefit will not work. It would be more realistic to assume the first five years yield zero net benefits, so benefits would only be expected in the sixth through the tenth year of the ten-year period. This produces a final figure—with all due caveats—of $500 million.

---

[9] Although no respondent said flatly this would occur, many (from AHIMA, AHA, HFMA, and two AAHP members, among others) stated they thought that it was likely.

Confidence Range: Again, many parameters are subject to alternative viewpoints. Some of them—e.g., the total money spent on claims adjudication, the assumption that the cost of processing a claim is proportional to the number of cycles it makes—could be refined with more data. However, these parameters are dominated by the big assumptions, notably the 1 percent reduction in the average number of cycles per claim and the assumption that net benefit becomes positive after five years. In this case, the reduction may well be as large as 3 to 5 percent, rather than 1 percent. We therefore use a wide range of $200 million to $2,500 million to represent this benefit.

Fewer Improper Claims

Concerning fraud, the WEDI report goes on to argue:

> If a new coding scheme were implemented, there would be increased opportunity for fraud in the beginning, when people are less familiar with the new codes. It might be more difficult to detect potential duplicates, unbundled services, or upcoding of procedures during the transition when two versions of code sets would be in effect. In the longer term, it is possible that fraud could be reduced since ICD-10-CM and ICD-10-PCS are more specific and there are fewer "gray" areas in coding. (p. 12)

Thus, WEDI claims that people who purport to perform a more complex procedure than they actually did would not be able to hide behind ambiguities in the code definition.[10]

A Benefits Scenario

Numbers similar to those in the last section can be applied to generating a scenario for the benefits of reduced abuse. Here the question is how much less abuse would take place because those potentially committing fraud can no longer hide behind ambiguities in the codes. Although the GAO has estimated an annual total of $13 billion in improper payments,[11] a large percentage of claims are probably matters of honest dispute, leaving the rest as matters of dishonesty. The assumption here is that some percentage of abusers, would, if confronted, blame the ambiguities in the code, therefore hoping to avoid penalties. Of those, some will see ICD-10 as making such an excuse harder. Some percentage of *them* will stop committing fraud; others will do so but find other ways of assuaging their fear of being caught. But one must also add something to accommodate the temptation to abuse the system hoping to get away with it in the initial confusion when the new codes are introduced. So, calculating benefits for ICD-10-CM requires knowing

F =   total cost of improper payments (as estimated above)

DH =   percentage of improper fraud due to abuse

---

[10] At first blush, the direct conversion from the patient record to a code would tend to make upcoding (fudging codes to rate a greater reimbursement) more difficult and thus rarer. But it also creates the risk that patient records themselves would be fudged for reimbursement purposes, thereby creating a misleading picture of the patient. This could confuse later physicians and perhaps lead to the wrong medical care.

[11] GAO, *Federal Budget,* "Opportunities for Oversight and Improved Use of Taxpayer Funds," Statement of David M. Walker, Comptroller General of the United States, GAO-03-922T.

P_{ambig} = percentage of abuse carried out by those who believe that the ambiguity of the old codes is enough of an excuse to keep them out of serious trouble

$P_{noambig}$ = percentage of *those* perpetrated by people who will see the clarity of the new codes as eliminating that excuse

$P_{nofraud}$ = percentage of people who stop abusing the system (rather than find a different excuse).

The calculation is therefore $F \times DH \times P_{ambig} \times P_{noambig} \times P_{nofraud}$, where $F \times DH$ is the total amount of fraud.

We start, as noted, with F = \$13 billion. We estimate DH to be 20 percent, but such a number is extremely soft. A large percentage of improper payments stems from honest disagreements about what proper cost and benefit coverage should be. Another large percentage comes from providers who code as they do in order to ensure that patients are covered for tests and procedures that they honestly believe are warranted but that may be questioned under existing rules. To say that \$2.5 billion (nearly 20 percent of \$13 billion) represents unambiguous theft may *seem* very high, but it is less than 0.2 percent of the total cost of health care in the United States and compares, in dollar amounts, to categories such as credit-card fraud or unpaid-for phone calls.

The next few estimates are offered for the sake of argument. We use a figure of 8 percent for P_{ambig}—the amount of abuse carried out by those who do so only because they believe they can claim code ambiguities if they are caught. This may seem low, but it represents the consequences of a third-order line of argument: Abusers have to imagine getting caught, and they have to imagine evading all or most of the consequences of getting caught through a convincing argument. Traditionally, third-order arguments play weak roles in criminal behavior.

We arbitrarily set the next two parameters, $P_{noambig}$ and $P_{nofraud}$, at 50 percent. That is, half of the abusers look at ICD-10-CM and ICD-10-PCS and conclude that hiding behind code ambiguities will no longer work and half of those who come to that conclusion find other fig leaves to hide behind; the other half decide to continue abusing the system.[12]

All these assumptions leave a benefit of \$50 million a year. To annualize this number over ten years, we make the same assumption that we did in the last calculation: the first five years net out because it takes that long for fraud prompted by the initial uncertainties of the new code to be offset by the reduced opportunities for fraud inherent in code ambiguities. Again, we count only the benefits accruing from the sixth through the tenth year. The final figure—with all due caveats—is \$250 million.

Confidence Range: Many judgment calls and assumptions went into this calculation. The most critical judgment call was in making distinctions among fraud, exaggeration, and legitimate differences of opinion. The most critical assumptions were in the many variables involved in collectively estimating what percentage of abusers (1) leveraged the ambiguities

---

[12] We argued earlier in this report that the elimination of outright fraud was an unambiguous benefit because one should not count the reduction in fraudulent payments as a cost to a provider. Conversely, a shift in payments over honest measures of interpretation cannot be counted as a net benefit. In between is a great gray area where providers give themselves the benefit of the doubt when coding and making claims. Is their reduced ability to do so a benefit without countervailing costs, or a benefit with equal and opposite costs? Our calculations take the latter view, but alternative viewpoints are not unreasonable.

of the code to cover their activities, (2) perceived that ICD-10-CM and ICD-10-PCS would reduce such ambiguities, and (3) would not find alternative ways of doing the same thing. Because a wide variation in this estimate is called for, we use a range of $100 million to $1,000 million to represent this benefit.

Better Understanding of the Value of New Procedures

Because most new procedures are currently lumped together with older ones, it is often difficult to discern the value and applicability of the new ones. ICD-10-PCS, by permitting much finer differentiation, permits these new procedures to be assessed—either by providers or by others.

Discharge statistics can be used by providers to evaluate their own health care competencies or by others to evaluate providers. Finer distinctions may permit more-precise evaluation. By analyzing its own cases, a provider could determine what procedures it does well relative to its peer institutions and where it falls behind. It can use such information to reallocate its resources and promote itself to referring physicians. Better codes for procedures, especially, aid this process.[13] Providers may want to go back to discover the results of using a particular technique or device; codes that include such detail make it easier to identify which records to pull in finding out this information.

Another way to exploit discharge procedures—associated with the Pacific Business Group on Health, among others—is to persuade payers to forward their claims data to a central clearinghouse. By aggregating each individual's inpatient and outpatient records, it is possible to get a more synoptic view of how successfully diseases and conditions are treated over time. Early data mining of treatments has generated some new conclusions about such procedures as coronary artery bypass graft surgery.

A Benefits Scenario

In estimating the value of research on procedures, we must keep several assumptions in mind. First, only a certain percentage of procedures (those that did not get their own code in ICD-9-CM, Volume 3) are likely to win *new* separate identification in ICD-10-PCS—and identifying them assumes correct coding. Second, insofar as the research is meant to affect decisions, we are looking at decisions to do the procedure more often (say, for a broader selection of patients) or less often (i.e., to consider alternative procedures in some cases or to quit doing the procedure). However, such research says little about *how* to do the procedure (except when two different ways of doing a procedure are identified as two different procedures in ICD-10-PCS and are therefore found to yield different outcomes). Needless to add, clinical practice is unlikely to follow research results immediately or totally. Third, many of these procedures are so well accepted that no feasible amount of research is likely to

---

[13] Gauging this benefit raises the following question: If more-detailed information is valuable, why does it take a new code to persuade providers to define what they need and go ahead and collect it? The most plausible answers to this question are (1) collection requires software that will not reach the market until the codes are made official, (2) the more-refined coding required to capture such information may be confused by coders with the codes required for payment, (3) the real benefits require that other providers, notably primary care physicians, provide better information on diagnoses, (4) what providers really want is information on other providers, and getting this requires a standard, and (5) even though better decision support cannot in itself justify greater data acquisition, it still may be an offsetting benefit.

affect the decision to undertake them. Fourth, research using ICD-10-PCS hospital discharge data is only one of many sources of information on such procedures. Payers, for instance, already have access to physician-based claims encoded in CPT. There will also be controlled studies that rely on information in patient records or conveyed directly by physicians. Last, and perhaps most important, are stories of failures and successes passed around among specialists.

So the variables we are interested in are

M = number of procedures performed each year that are separately identified from their larger group only in ICD-10-PCS and are sufficiently different from the procedures with which they were earlier identified to suggest that they offer different outcomes

$P_{doneenough}$ = percentage of such procedures that are performed often enough to yield a basis for statistically significant difference in outcomes

$P_{ICDresearch}$ = odds that research using ICD-10-PCS discharge statistics says something about the applicability of such procedures that are missed by other methods (e.g., controlled studies)

P_{DELM} = percentage change in the number[14] of procedures done as a result of ICD-10-PCS–based research

B = average benefit of either doing the procedure when it otherwise would not have been done or vice versa.

Therefore, the value of greater knowledge on the efficacy and appropriateness of new procedures is $M \times P_{doneenough} \times P_{ICDresearch} \times P_{DELM} \times B$.

To fill in this scenario, we will use numbers comparable to the ones in the section on more-accurate payments for new procedures.

In that section, we used a term of 200,000 significantly new inpatient procedures a year (here, "significantly" is indicated by the willingness of proponents to ask CMS to find a new code for them). In this scenario, we will have five years' worth of new procedures to research when ICD-10-PCS comes into effect and 15 years' worth ten years later, for an average of ten years' worth or 2 million. As in the section on more-accurate payments for new procedures, we remove 40 percent as important enough to have gotten their own codes in ICD-9-CM, Volume 3. This leaves 1.2 million procedures a year as the subject of research.

We then assume that one-third of all such procedures are so specialized that statistical analysis of hospital discharge records is unlikely to reveal anything of statistical significance. That is, $P_{doneenough}$ = 2/3, leaving 800,000 procedures a year.

The next parameter, $P_{ICDresearch}$, is likely to be low because it represents the combined odds that (1) a procedure is misapplied (i.e., it should be performed on more,

---

[14] This is an absolute number that may be positive even if the number of procedures done does not change. It is the sum of those who get the procedure thanks to new knowledge, or who do not get the procedure thanks to new knowledge. Economic theory suggests that the average benefit for each such patient is proportional to the number of procedures that are changed as a result of better knowledge on the procedure's outcome.

fewer, and/or different patients), (2) this fact has escaped notice through all previous ways of knowing such facts, but (3) the procedure becomes the subject of research based on analyzing ICD-10-PCS codes, as a result of which (4) such misapplication is discovered and credibly received. Given these combined odds, we use a figure of 4 percent, leaving 32,000 procedures a year.

We then estimate the average number of procedure incident changes at 0.5. That is, for every 10 patients who would have received the procedure prior to such research, we can identify five patients for whom the procedure is now contraindicated but hitherto indicated, or now indicated but hitherto contraindicated. So 16,000 procedures are shifted. Finally, we use the same $5,000 net benefit for B as in the section on more-accurate payments for new procedures. This produces a final figure—with all due caveats—of $800 million (16,000 × $5,000 × 10 years).

Confidence Range: Several hard-to-quantify assumptions went into this estimate. Some were carried over from the section on more-accurate payments for new procedures. Others represent the extra knowledge that would be gained from an analysis of ICD-10-CM records that are not otherwise available from extant sources, and the effect of extra knowledge on the distribution of who received which procedures. Adding further uncertainty is the likelihood that most of the benefits are likely to come from the knowledge gained from a relatively small handful of procedures—but we have no good way of knowing in advance what those procedures will be. We therefore use a range of $100 million to $1,500 million to represent this benefit.

Improved Disease Management

Disease management is the process by which HMOs and other care management organizations work with patients—especially those with chronic conditions such as diabetes, asthma, and heart disease—to ensure that they are receiving the correct quality of care, reminders for treatment, and referrals to classes and other self-management techniques. If disease management is successful, it can postpone or eliminate the risk of the more serious complications that send people to hospitals. By permitting more-specific coding of patient conditions, it may be possible for care management organizations to identify which members require disease management and to tailor programs more precisely to their conditions, thereby raising the efficacy of disease management and saving both lives and money.

Admittedly, disease management services can be performed by primary care physicians (who rely on personal knowledge of or detailed notes on patients rather than on discharge codes). Yet many patients either lack a primary care physician or have many physicians, no one of whom is responsible for managing the patient. Care management organizations may usefully back up primary care physicians, identified as such. Since much of the work of disease management—finding eligible patients, sending them reminders, giving them information—can be automated, care management organizations can run algorithms through patient records en masse to identify patients who need disease management and deliver such management automatically. For example, one large payer sends out a million alerts a year.

The potential benefits of disease management are large. Diabetes, for example, is a chronic condition whose prevalence in the population is increasing. It accounts for over

60,000 deaths annually and many more severe and costly complications that, with better management, might be reduced as a result of more detailed diagnostic[15] information. Nevertheless, our expectations should be tempered by the following considerations:

- Many primary care physicians do not use the specificity that already exists in the existing ICD-9-CM codes. It is unclear whether they will react to a more specific set of codes by using distinctions that were previously unused. Other physicians produce diagnostic codes that indicate not the underlying cause of the encounter (e.g., diabetes) but its proximate cause (e.g., kidney dysfunction). One respondent has suggested that some of the differentiations in diabetes (e.g., neuropathy) exceed what is typically recorded in doctors' notes.

- Many care management organizations, as a result, use other indicators to differentiate diabetic patients from one another: HbA1c tests and diagnostic codes for co-morbidities.

- At least one large HMO is getting away from classification codes altogether, using instead the more highly refined information available from a standard nomenclature system: Systematized Nomenclature of Human and Veterinary Medicine—Clinical Terms (SNOMED-CT).

- Conversely, a larger percentage, perhaps half, of all the screening that is done to determine suitability for disease management uses relatively broad episode treatment groups (ETGs), the most popular set of which has 500 to 1,000 groups. Such data are more highly aggregated than the ICD-9 codes, let alone ICD-10. The more sophisticated algorithms use a mixture of diagnoses, procedures, laboratory tests, and medications to determine what condition the patient has and, thus, whether disease management is warranted. The finer details available from ICD-10 cannot hurt the implementation of this algorithm, but responses to date do not suggest they will contribute much more accuracy to such determinations.

A Benefits Scenario

ICD-10-CM could conceivably help disease management in two ways: (1) better identifying who should receive disease management services, and (2) tailoring disease management more precisely to those identified. We estimate the benefits of each separately.

We assume that the more detailed information resulting from ICD-10-CM diagnostic codes will result in a better selection of patients, where *better* means more likely to profit

---

[15] ICD-9-CM has 40 diabetes codes based on (1) whether the diabetes is Type 1 or Type 2, (2) whether it is controlled or uncontrolled, and (3) possible complications: (a) none, (b) ketoacidosis, (c) hyperosmolarity, (d) other coma, (e) renal, (f) opthalmic, (g) neurological, (h) circulatory, (i) other, or (j) unknown. ICD-10-CM has 208 potential diabetes codes (six types of diabetes multiplied by 35 ways to express complications but without the two codes for Type 1 diabetes w/hyperosmolarity). The differences from ICD-9-CM are the following: (a) The controlled versus uncontrolled distinction has been eliminated. (b) Two new categories were added: drug-induced diabetes, and diabetes due to underlying condition together with "other" and "unknown." (c) The three categories of complications—ketoacidosis, hyperosmolarity, and other coma—have been changed to ketoacidosis with or without coma, and hyperosmolarity with and without coma. (d) Renal has been expanded to nephropathy, Ebstien's disease, renal failure, and other renal complications. (e) Opthalmic has been expanded to background retinopathy, proliferative retinopathy, cataracts, other, and unknown. (f) Neurologic has been expanded to mononeuropathy, polyneuropathy, autonomic polyneuropathy, other, and unknown. (g) Circulatory complications are with or without gangrene. (h) Some other complications with their subcategories are to be separately identified: arthropathy (neurologic or non-neurologic), dermatitis (foot ulcer, skin ulcer, other, or unknown), oral (periodontal or not), hypoglycemia (with or without coma), and hyperglycemia.

from closer oversight. For this to happen, the patient must be covered by a plan (1) that has a disease management program, (2) where selection into a program uses ICD codes as a key variable, (3) where the details from ICD-10-CM can make a difference, so that (4) patients otherwise not in the program are pulled inside. As a result of disease management, patients' indicators (notably HbA1c)—and therefore their quality of life—improve. So the inputs are

D = number of diabetics

P_{dmp} = percentage of diabetics covered by payers with disease management programs

P_{dm} = percentage of covered diabetics in disease management

P_{icd} = percentage of disease management programs that use ICD codes as their primary means of looking for participants

$P_{bettericd}$ = percentage of patients outside disease management whose ICD information is improved

$P_{bettericdin}$ = ratio of those who are added to the program as a result of better ICD information

$P_{betteroff}$ = percentage of those added to the program as a result of better ICD statistics, who, as a result of the program, reduce their parameters (defined as HbA1c scores) below some threshold (lower is defined as better)

Q = gains per patient from staying below the threshold for a year.

The calculation is $D \times P_{dmp} \times (1 - P_{dm}) \times P_{dm} \times P_{bettericd} \times P_{bettericdin} \times P_{betteroff} \times Q$. Up to the last character, the formula calculates the number of affected patients.

There are two types of diabetics for purposes of this calculation: those who have been diabetic since childhood (500,000) and those who acquired diabetes late in life (roughly 10,000,000). Because the potential benefits of disease management are so much greater for those in the first category—largely because, being younger, they would otherwise expect to have more years to live, the running numbers total will be stated as 500,000/10 million.

We further estimate that 60 percent of diabetics are covered by payers with disease management programs (P_{dmp}) but half of those patients are *not* in disease management programs (P_{dm}) of one sort or another—hence, 150,000/3,000,000 people. Of these programs, half use ETGs to sort out their patients, and we assume that two-thirds of the remainder use ICD codes as their primary sorting device (P_{icd} = 1/3). This leaves 50,000/1,000,000 people whose management could be improved by better ICD codes.

At this point in the calculation, we concentrate on the one million adult diabetics on the theory that those whose diabetes started in childhood are already well identified. In contrast, as many as one-third of those with adult-onset diabetes have not even been diagnosed.

The next parameter, $P_{bettericdin}$, reflects the likelihood that the most-detailed ICD-10-CM codes are used and that these one million patients have conditions that would be coded differently (i.e., with more specificity) in ICD-10-CM compared with how they are coded in ICD-9-CM. Since there are grounds for pessimism on the first likelihood and grounds for skepticism on the second, we estimate that ICD-10-CM would actually reveal new information for about 20 percent, or 200,000 people.

We then assume that half of these 200,000 people enter into disease management programs as a result of more-specific information ($P_{bettericdin}$). Of these 100,000, roughly one-fifth improve their indicators[16] past a given threshold[17] and thereby enjoy the equivalent of an extra half-year of full-quality life,[18] the value of which we evaluate at $50,000 per year.[19] Thus, the total benefit from putting the right people into disease management is $500 million.

The calculations for the second part of the benefit scenario use the same parameters as the first part of the calculation—that is, 500,000/10 million for those whose payers have disease management programs, 150,000/3 million for those who *are* in such programs (because this time we are looking for people whose programs are adjusted because of finer ICD scores), 50,000/1 million for those whose payers use ICD as the key decision variable, and 5,000/100,000 for those whose condition is better understood because of more-specific ICD-based data. This 5,000/100,000 is then multiplied by:

$P_{betterplan}$ = percentage of people whose disease management plan is changed as a result of more precise ICD information

$P_{betteroff2}$ = percentage of people whose parameters are improved past some threshold thanks to being more precisely managed.

Here, the full calculation is: $D \times P_{dmp} \times P_{dm} \times P_{icd} \times P_{bettericd} \times P_{betterplan} \times P_{betteroff2} \times Q$.

Since this is a scenario, we will use similar numbers throughout the rest of the calculation. We assume $P_{betterplan}$ to be 50 percent (because knowing something more about a patient and adjusting a program based on this knowledge are two different things), but the assumption that a more refined program will improve health enough to move someone past a threshold is only 10 percent in this case (that is, the gain from putting someone into a program is roughly twice as great as the gain from adjusting the program). In this case, however, we assume that those with childhood-onset diabetes gain two extra years of quality life while the rest gain six months.[20] Thus, 50 people get the extra two years of life, for a benefit of $50 million; 10,000 get an extra six months of life, for a benefit of $250 million—with a grand total of $300 million.

Finally, we assume that two-thirds of the benefits that ICD-10 offers to disease management accrue to diabetics and the rest to everyone else, so that we multiply $800

---

[16]See, for example, C. Barr Taylor et al., "Evaluation of a Nurse-Care Management System to Improve Outcomes in Patients with Complicated Diabetes," *Diabetes Care,* Vol. 26, 2003, pp. 1058–1063.

[17] This is a first-order approximation used to facilitate calculation. It is more likely that more people will improve, but not as much. Rather than measuring well-being on every point of the continuum, we can get roughly the same benefit totals by counting only those who cross a threshold and comparing the average well-being of those under the threshold with the average of those over the threshold.

[18] The assumption that people enjoy two years of full-quality life because their condition deteriorates more slowly is really a first-order-approximation way of describing two curves of quality-of-life deterioration that are separated by two years.

[19] This $50,000 also includes the avoided costs of treating people because they are healthier.

[20] To reiterate footnote 17, this calculation is a proxy for smaller gains enjoyed by more people.

million (the benefits of being able to manage diabetes better) by 1.5. Because this calculation represents a cumulative benefit over a total patient population, it does not have to be multiplied to produce a ten-year number. The final figure—with all due caveats—is thus $1.2 billion.

Confidence Range: Several estimates and assumptions went into this figure. Because they link serially, modest variations in each of them can lead to major variations when they are multiplied together. The key estimate is the number of patients whose conditions are screened using ICD-10-CM discharge data. The most important assumptions relate to (1) how much more information is available from ICD-10-CM, (2) the extent to which such information changes a disease management program, and (3) the gains possible with those programs. Disease management is a relatively young field that is still growing, so our knowledge of how effective it is remains provisional. We therefore use a wide range of $200 million to $1,500 million to represent this benefit.

Better Understanding of Health Conditions and Health Care Outcomes

The tens of millions of annual hospital discharge records constitute a database of enormous potential in assessing both the nation's health and the relationship between health care and outcomes.[21] If the diagnoses and procedures were more finely specified, the benefits for third-party[22] research could only improve. The ability to discover previously hidden relationships or even uncover phenomena early (e.g., incipient epidemics) can be of potentially enormous value. For instance, knowing whether and in what circumstances laparoscopic surgery improves health outcomes more than does open surgery could affect thousands of lives and save billions of dollars.

Indeed, the greater detail of ICD-10-CM and ICD-10-PCS, coupled with the prospects that the cleaner logic of the codes may lead to fewer coding errors in the long term, cannot help but improve research. One should never discount the possibility of a breakthrough research finding that could carry enormously positive ramifications for better health and/or improved economics. Nevertheless, guarded optimism is called for, rather than unrestrained optimism.

The analysis of codes is an essential component of research in which there is no direct access to patient medical records. Yet studies that infer conclusions from hospital discharge statistics (also known as "uncontrolled studies") sit at one end of the spectrum of analytic techniques. At the other end are controlled studies in which researchers select protocols and specifically code diagnoses and procedures for analysis. In between are studies in which patients and protocols are not selected, but diagnoses and procedures are specifically accounted for. Furthermore, although finer distinctions have their merits in doing analysis, the additional distinctions have to be those that make a difference. And even if they do make

---

[21] The most comprehensive public database on hospital discharges is the Healthcare Cost and Utilization Project (HCUP) from the U.S. Agency for Healthcare Research and Quality (AHRQ). As of May 2003, the Nationwide Inpatient Sample contained data on five to eight million hospital stays from about 1,000 surveyed hospitals. There are also private data consolidators with similar information: e.g., University HealthSystem Consortium, Premier, CHCHA, Solucient. Solucient has access to HCUP data plus data it receives from payer organizations; it claims a database of roughly 20 million records, but the records are not publicly accessible.

[22] As distinguished from research done by providers or payers on data from their patients or members.

a difference, the gains from fine distinctions are often vitiated by the smaller population sizes within each category, which erode statistical significance. Last, long-range studies may require some reliable means of translating pre-transition diagnoses and procedures to make them compatible with post-transition diagnoses and procedures in order to permit comparisons over time.

A specific problem with hospital discharge datasets, at least for third-party researchers, is the difficulty of determining exactly what happened to the patients after they were discharged from the hospital. One can tell if patients died during their stay but not if they died the day after they were discharged. Because hospital records are typically provided without names, one cannot even determine if patients reentered the same hospital a week later with the same or a different condition. Information on the quality of life for such patients is even harder to capture. Granted, a few privileged researchers *can* get access to health data with health identification claim (HIC) numbers, which at least permits one hospital stay to be correlated with another. Access to such data, however, is managed by the U.S. Agency for Healthcare Research and Quality (AHRQ). Access is easily granted only to AHRQ employees and requires that the analysis be done only on certain specific machines (in other words, the data cannot leave the premises). Few AHRQ researchers work with the data, perhaps as a reaction to the earlier and unwarranted optimism about what such data could tell researchers. Outsiders can get the data if AHRQ approves, but AHRQ rules require that no data be left behind on researcher computers—something difficult to guarantee. Consequently, very few outsiders use the data.

Dr. Lisa Iezzoni has observed that ICD-10-CM codes have the potential to reveal a good deal more about quality of care, so that the data could be used in a more meaningful way to enable better understanding of complications, better designing of clinically robust algorithms, and better tracking of the outcomes of care. Nevertheless, most research agglomerates information in specific categories into supercategories, not only to create statistically significant sample sizes but also to avoid the misleading effect of minor coding errors or of coders unwilling or unable to make the fine distinctions that ICD-9 already allows. Indeed, some software companies specialize in grouper software precisely to support providers engaged in such analysis. True, a finer, more scientifically precise, set of distinctions is likely to determine which diagnoses or procedures are grouped together. Such distinctions cannot but help improve analyses—but only somewhat.

Another constraint that limits the value of added specificity is the prevalence of coding errors and the likelihood that, as more distinctions are called for and more differentiation has to be made (i.e., is it this or that?), more—albeit smaller—errors will creep in. As long as errors are random, they are unlikely to create spurious findings, but they do tend to throw into doubt findings that would otherwise arise from the data.

At least two researchers say the new codes may get in the way of research. When codes change, it becomes harder to compare data over time.[23] But this difficulty should not be exaggerated because crosswalks can be applied to the new data to make them comparable to the old (little, of course, can be done to old data to go back and capture the differentiations that could have been recorded if the new codes had been in use). Although, as noted, ICD-10-CM is not a one-to-many expansion of ICD-9-CM, to the extent that aggregation is

---

[23] See Betty Grigg et al., "Coding Changes and Apparent HIV/AIDS Mortality Trends in Florida, 1999," *Journal of the American Medical Association,* Vol. 286, No. 15, 2001, p. 1839.

preserved and discarded distinctions are now believed to be unimportant or misleading, a crosswalk may be good enough for most purposes.

Nevertheless, greater specificity has to be rated a good thing on net. Exactly what we will learn from greater specificity is hard to forecast with any confidence, but such uncertainty typifies all serious research.

Enhanced Ability to Evaluate Providers

Better data should help payers rate providers. Payers (compared with outside researchers) have the benefit of having continuing and comprehensive data on their own members. This benefit allows them to link one hospital stay to the next, as well as to outpatient visits and associated laboratory tests. One payer indicated that it was working to make such ratings public (via the Web) and use them to create, over time, what would be a top tier of providers within its overall preferred provider listing. Patients would be steered to providers that offered cost-effective health care. Here, better codes permit more precise and informative distinctions.

Again, the value of more precise codes needs to be put into perspective. Although the specificity of ICD-10-PCS is much greater than the specificity of ICD-9-CM Volume 3, it is not the only information available to payers, and thus the proper basis of comparison is between ICD-10-PCS plus other information (some of which offers differentiating detail missing in ICD-9-CM Volume 3) and ICD-9-CM Volume 3 plus other information.[24]

Where would one use greater specificity in analyzing providers? One could analyze their relative ability to undertake procedures or to respond to diagnoses that previously were lumped in with others. But the problem of statistical significance is much more severe when rating providers, no one of which accounts for more than 3 percent of the total patient population. One might choose to aggregate all new procedures (i.e., those previously lumped in with old procedures) for analysis. That would generate new—and perhaps statistically significant—data, but whether it would yield a meaningful indicator of performance is unclear. It is also possible that finer diagnostic and procedural codes could be used to better norm the patients whom providers treat (otherwise, providers who treat sicker patients would falsely appear to perform worse than average). But ICD-10-CM's contribution to indicating severity is, at best, modest.

There is also the question of how well one can rate providers based on data generated by the providers themselves. The coding of diagnoses, in particular, has discretionary elements. It is subject to interpretation and has been known to shift over time. Twenty years of history[25] suggest that DRGs do creep upward (from less serious and resource-intensive to more serious and resource-intensive) to justify higher reimbursement rates—even after demographics, such as an aging population, are accounted for. New York and California have tried to get providers to indicate whether a particular patient condition was acquired after admission to the hospital; at least in New York State, such information has been

---

[24] Other information includes physicians' claims forms coded in CPT-4 and received by payers. CPT-4 has greater specificity than does ICD-9-CM, Volume 3.

[25] Grace M. Carter and Paul B. Ginsburg, *The Medicare Case Mix Index Increase: Medical Practice Changes, Aging, and DRG Creep*, Santa Monica, Calif.: RAND Corporation, R-3292-HCFA, 1985.

inconsistently reported.[26] In a study of discectomy patients,[27] Drs. Romano et al. concluded that "ICD-9-CM complications were underreported . . . especially at hospitals with low risk-adjusted complication rates." Further muddying the waters is the rate of errors that are commonly encountered in coding.[28] If randomly distributed, such errors are more likely to lead to reduced statistical certainty and only rarely to spurious conclusions. But even after people get used to ICD-10, there is ample reason to believe that the number of errors will rise. Although the errors may be smaller (confusing fine distinctions) rather than larger (crossing broader categories), they tend to dilute the value of finer information.

We therefore conclude that the contribution of ICD-10-CM and ICD-10–PCS to rating providers is likely to be modest but positive.

Timelier Intervention for Emergent Diseases

It is theoretically possible that more-precise disease categorization, coupled with the timely reporting of diseases, could permit the public health community to detect emergent diseases (including deliberately induced ones) more rapidly than it does now and to contain them before they get out of hand. The potential benefits are enormous. If better diagnostic codes could improve the odds of heading off the next SARS-like disease, even by a few percentage points, the switch could pay for itself many times over through that benefit alone (SARS is said to have cost the Asian economy alone well in excess of $10 billion[29]). Similar benefits may come from being able to spot clusters of diseases that might be traced to environmental or occupational conditions. There is some indication that the ability to differentiate diseases more finely may help analysts spot unusual patterns that would otherwise be lost in the broader averages.[30] That noted, ICD-10-CM was not designed for syndromic surveillance, and access to hospital discharge records would have to be accelerated to provide for timely

---

[26] Interview with Robert Davis, April 21, 2003.

[27] Patrick Romano et al., "Can Administrative Data Be Used to Compare Postoperative Complication Rates Across Hospitals?" *Medical Care*, Vol. 40, No. 10, 2002, pp. 856–867.

[28] See, e.g., Daniel A. Ollendorf et al., "Is Sepsis Accurately Coded on Hospital Bills?" *Value in Health*, Vol. 5, No. 2, 2002, 79–81:

> While [administrative] datasets are readily accessible and relatively inexpensive . . . the sensitivity of coded diagnoses from health-care claims data has been reported to be below 80% overall, ranging from 58% for peripheral vascular disease to over 90% for several types of cancer. . . . Our findings indicate that the use of ICD-9-CM codes for identifying patients with sepsis is only moderately sensitive and may miss up to one-quarter of patients with this disease. . . . Hospital information systems typically include 15 to 20 diagnosis codes for each admission, while the UB-92 format allows for only 9 codes. It is possible that, for some patients, sepsis was coded on the medical record but not on the hospital bill. We believe that this accounts for a relatively small percentage of cases because sepsis is considered a modifying diagnosis (i.e., one that may increase payment under Medicare's Prospective Payment System) and is therefore likely to appear on most hospital bills.

The problem is not limited to the United States. As Dr. S. Schulz et al. observed in "Conversion Problems Concerning Automated Mapping from ICD-10 to ICD-9," *Methods of Information in Medicine*, Vol. 37, 1998, pp. 254–259, "We are aware of the mediocre quality of codification in clinical practice at least in Germany. If one must always take into account a certain amount of doubtful codes, a too rigid approach to a conversion table would not be adequate."

[29] "The Cost of SARS: $11 Billion and Rising," *Far Eastern Economic Review*, Vol. 166, No. 16, 2003, p. 12.

[30] As argued both by Gail Graham of the Veterans' Administration and by the health information management director of a major hospital corporation.

intervention in the case of a fast-moving epidemic. We therefore conclude that ICD-10-CM, in its present form, is unlikely to contribute much in this area.

Summary of Benefits

Table 3.1 summarizes those benefits for which we could generate numbers. It indicates the relevant category, a scenario-based benefit estimate, and the code (ICD-10-CM or ICD-10-PCS) to which these benefits can primarily be ascribed. The total is $700 million on the low end to $7,700 million on the high end.

Table 3.1
Summary of Estimated Benefits over a Ten-Year Period[a]

Category	Benefit ($ million)	Largely Due to
More-accurate payment for new procedures	100–1,200	ICD-10-PCS
Fewer rejected claims	200–2,500	both
Fewer fraudulent claims	100–1,000	both
Better understanding of new procedures	100–1,500	ICD-10-PCS
Improved disease management	200–1,500	ICD-10-CM

[a] Benefits are not discounted over time.

CHAPTER FOUR

Simultaneous Versus Sequential Switching

If switching to *both* ICD-10-CM and ICD-10-PCS is warranted, is it better to do both at once or one after the other? Many witnesses to the NCVHS and many we interviewed shuddered at the thought of trying to implement new codes before they had finished complying with HIPAA requirements. But no one who testified or whom we interviewed suggested that it was better to implement the code switch sequentially.[1] Canada, which also implemented changes for both diagnoses and procedures, did them together.

Switching both at once makes sense for several reasons. One is psychological: It is easier to get people (e.g., coders) mentally prepared for a change in their lives once rather than twice. If students and even teachers have to travel to be trained, they need do so only once. Similarly, it is easier to review a complex billing system to look for where ICD-9-CM, Volumes 1, 2, and 3 are used than it is to do the same procedure twice: first for Volumes 1 and 2, then a year later for Volume 3. The same is true for testing: Simultaneous change means testing only once rather than twice.[2] Dealing with transition issues, such as getting through the errors of miscoding or misinterpreting until everyone is used to the new system, is also better done all at once rather than in two periods separated by months or a year. People can focus attention and resources on the process of making a smooth changeover and getting the new system down pat—leaving only a few individuals to work on residual problems.

The last rationale for simultaneity is the construction of DRGs and other eligibility and payments logic. They are determined by both diagnoses identified and procedures performed. Although, as noted above, CMS does not expect to alter the logic of DRG determination right after ICD-10 is implemented, there is little doubt that the added specificity of the diagnoses and the greater number of procedures identified separately will give considerable impetus to altering DRGs, once people become used to the new codes. A sequential transition to ICD-10 would postpone that process. The same, more or less, would be the case for payers' eligibility and reimbursement determinations. In both cases, it is best to consider the impact of new diagnoses and procedures together.

Table 4.1 takes Table 2.1 and adds further costs for making a sequential switch. At the high end, these costs are composed of

---

[1] One person who testified suggested switching to ICD-10-CM as a trial to help determine whether the more difficult switch to ICD-10-PCS would cost too much.

[2] This assumes that most tests can be done in one pass because serious errors will be rare. This is not the case if serious errors are common or if errors in implementing ICD-10-CM and ICD-10-PCS interact with one another. In that case, tests would have to be run multiple times anyway, and there would be little advantage to changing both codes together.

Table 4.1
Additional Estimated Costs of a Sequential Switch

	Personnel	Cost Estimate ($ million)	Additional Costs ($ million)
Training	Full-time coders	100–150	0–20
	Part-time coders	50–150	
	Code users	25–50	0–10
	Physicians	25–100	
Productivity losses	Coders	0–150[a]	
	Physicians	50–250 [a]	
System changes	Providers	50–200	5–50
	Software vendors	50–125	5–20
	Payers	100–250	5–50
	CMS	25–125	5–20

[a] Total over ten years.

- running separate training sessions for ICD-10-PCS and ICD-10-CM instead of doing them together
- conducting systems integration twice rather than once, for ICD-10-CM and then ICD-10-PCS (or vice versa)
- for some payers, developing interim logic algorithms for evaluating "medical necessity."

The low-end figure of $20 million reflects the possibility that people will act as if the second switch to the ICD-10 version of the code (e.g., to ICD-10-PCS) is inevitable when the first (e.g., to ICD-10-CM) is promulgated. However, even if people decided to switch to both together when they only have to switch one at a time, there still remains the cost of building and using systems that can deal with one old and one new code simultaneously.

CHAPTER FIVE

Conclusions

Our analysis of costs and benefits has generated figures that indicate the following:

- Costs are expected to range between $425 million and $1.15 billion, plus $5 million to $40 million a year in lost productivity (with an additional $20 million to $170 million in costs if codes are switched sequentially).
- Benefits are expected to range between $700 million and $7.7 billion.

A broader perspective, however, may be in order. At almost a trillion and a half dollars, the U.S. health care industry is enormous. A small percentage shift in its efficacy or efficiency could easily swamp cost estimates that would amount to hundreds or millions of dollars. Nearly every other industry has found that if it wants a program of continuous process improvement, it has to start by measuring inputs and, particularly, outputs. Only after such measurement can alternatives be systematically compared.

The health care sector has lagged other industries in this approach, leaving great room for improvement. As such, codes—or at least the data contained in those codes—are central to the measurement process and hence to the goal of continuous process improvement. Anything that improves the codes—provided they contribute to good measurement—cannot help but have positive long-term ramifications.

All this suggests, however, that we know both what to measure to improve outcomes and how to measure it. Many people we talked to had done quite a bit of thinking on this score. Patient safety advocates laud the aforementioned "present-on-arrival" adjunct to diagnoses now collected by hospitals in California and New York (one proponent of ICD-10-PCS even went so far as to prefer having this indicator instead of ICD-10-PCS). Those who measure patient quality of care are interested in whether providers comply with HEDIS standards (e.g., are ACE-inhibitors and/or beta-blockers given to heart attack patients within their first 30 minutes in emergency rooms?). Others have noted that they would find indicators that differentiated diagnoses by severity to be quite useful. One researcher complained, in tracking septicemia, that there was only one code for urinary tract infections NEC (which mixes the kidney, the bladder, and the urethra), conflating a condition that is potentially fatal (urosepsis) and a condition that merely indicates the presence of some pathogen somewhere.[1] In many cases, severity can be directly indicated through laboratory test results (e.g., HbA1c for diabetes).

---

[1] In actuality, there are codes in ICD-9-CM for urinary tract infections caused by such infectious organisms as candida (112.2), diplococcus (098.0), and trichomonas (131.0).

Overall, there are good grounds for believing that the benefits are likely to exceed the initial break-in costs within a few years of code adoption. ICD-10 permits a considerable expansion in what we can know about the health of the population and the care it receives. The extent to which this information will be properly and intelligently exploited is hard to gauge at present. But the potential gain is large if the opportunities are taken.

CHAPTER SIX

Elements of a Transition Strategy

If the decision is made to implement ICD-10-CM and ICD-10-PCS, several steps would facilitate the transition:

1. Retain the practice of selecting a certain date by which everyone must make the transition. Everything associated with discharges on or before a given date would be submitted in ICD-9-CM; anything later, in ICD-10-CM and ICD-10-PCS. This would avoid having institutions keep two sets of books any longer than it takes to resolve old reimbursement claims.

2. Allow enough time for the transition. The consensus is that two to three years is appropriate, and it is understood that a year will probably be required between the time a decision to switch is made and the time that decision is cleared through the approvals process.

3. Prepare and promulgate a reliable and readily understandable crosswalk between ICD-9-CM and ICD-10-CM/ICD-10-PCS. Both payers and providers are relying on such a crosswalk as a way of bootstrapping themselves into the new codes and, in some cases, as a way of easing their transition into the new standard. Although the practice of translating every ICD-10-CM or ICD-10- PCS code into ICD-9-CM for processing is not a viable long-term strategy, it will permit users to postpone major systems changes until such changes can be scheduled to accommodate multiple requirements (rather than redoing a system for every new requirement).

4. Give serious thought to having a major provider code diagnoses and procedures in both ICD-9-CM and ICD-10-CM/ICD-10-PCS to determine which codes are interpreted similarly. This process would help to develop a crosswalk between ICD-9-CM and ICD-10-CM/ICD-10-PCS in practice as well as in theory. It would also help analysts who work with time series interpret before-and-after changes in health statistics.

Background Material

This appendix contains background material in three areas: how codes are used, how ICD-10-CM and ICD-10-PCS differ from their predecessors, and some issues involved in mapping from one code to another.

How Codes Are Used

ICD codes were invented to record how people died so that public knowledge about the health of the population could be improved. Starting in 1948, WHO extended the scope of ICD to include nonfatal diseases, indicating its understanding that the codes would be used for recording morbidity, thus enabling public health officials to begin to gauge the prevalence of conditions that were nonfatal but serious enough to require treatment.

With the rise of health insurance in the United States over the past half-century, these codes were also adopted as the primary mechanism for billing and reimbursement. Physicians and hospitals filled out reimbursement forms (e.g., HCFA-1500 for physicians, UB-92 for hospitals) that indicated one or more diagnostic conditions and whatever procedures were performed. Not every claim is honored. A key criterion for whether a medical procedure is paid for is whether it is "medically necessary" in light of the patient's diagnosis and condition. Insurance plans differ greatly over which diagnoses and conditions they cover, for which procedures they pay, and how much they pay. Most payers run very complex algorithms to determine "medical necessity"; such algorithms use codes as inputs. Changing the codes would necessitate changing at least some of the algorithms (and hence is a cost to be considered in a cost-benefit analysis).

Although most reimbursement processes pay for each procedure (and thus use procedure codes directly), almost all Medicare and many Medicaid claims are paid as a lump sum per encounter for inpatient services. The amount is based on which DRG the hospitalization best fits—based on the patient's diagnoses, procedures performed, and, in some cases, age and sex. More than 500 DRGs have been defined to capture the resources that a particular case requires, on the theory that many different but related procedures can be considered of comparable complexity. Within any DRG, whether the hospital does more or less work redounds to the hospital's gain or loss; generally, CMS will not pay more or less as a result.

Any sufficiently major change in classifying diagnoses and procedures is bound eventually to change how the DRGs are defined (indeed, 3M Health Information Systems, which developed ICD-10-PCS, is CMS's prime contractor for DRG definition and maintenance). Changing from one code set to another means that certain hospital visits that would have been classified with one DRG can be more correctly classified in another DRG. In the short run, however, CMS intends to fit the new codes into existing DRGs as best it can and give users some breathing room before making further changes.

Canada and Australia use a DRG concept to manage their single-payer systems. The Canadian province of Ontario found that when it adopted the Canadian version of ICD-10, it had to redefine 30 percent of its 470 case-mix groups. One out of seven cases shifted from one CMG to another as a result.

A Typical Life Cycle for Codes

Figure A.1 illustrates a life cycle for both diagnostic and procedure codes. It describes the creation and use of codes and suggests where the costs and benefits of new codes are likely to be found.[1] In the figure, the questions that describe costs are underscored; the questions that describe benefits are not. This distinction is a qualified one, however. It assumes that productivity will decline (a cost) and that the only question is, By how much? Similarly, it assumes that fewer claims will be sent back to the provider for more information and that the only question is, How many? But these are just assumptions. The reality could be more complex. For instance, productivity may first fall and then exceed what was experienced with ICD-9.

In the figure, the flow of information starts on the left with the patient record, which provides a detailed description of the patient's condition and what care was delivered in response.

When the patient's bill is prepared (usually at discharge time), this record is analyzed and codes are extracted from the information provided.[2] Generally speaking, physicians will know critical details of their patients' conditions that may not be apparent from the records they create. Although some physicians are familiar with the codes, they are unlikely to do the coding themselves (indeed, professional coders often urge that physicians not try, inasmuch as they are unlikely to be current on the annual code changes). Typically, hospitals and the larger physicians' clinics have specialized coders to do the extraction. In smaller office environments, coding is done by nurses and clerks. Physicians are occasionally consulted in the process, but they rarely do the actual coding.

Analysis of this record by a coder yields one or more diagnostic codes and procedure codes (not all cases will have procedure codes). This analysis effectively *compresses* the information by retaining the important features (or at least features important to its subsequent uses) and disregarding those features deemed less important.

---

[1] Given the varied contexts of health care in the United States, this figure typifies most, but not all, interactions. It is not meant to apply to long-term care facilities, home health care, or medical facilities such as some HMOs, which do not bill separately for individual encounters.

[2] In the outpatient setting, particularly in physicians' offices, this process is often more informal; e.g., the doctor may hand the patient record to a clerk with a succinct statement of the diagnosis and procedure.

Figure A.1
The Creation and Use of Codes

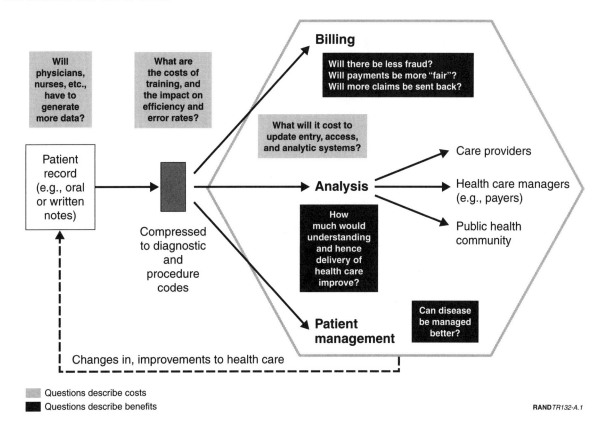

The retained information is almost always used in billing. Payers, in turn, analyze the various codes and charges and determine whether (1) the charges are to be paid, (2) the charges are to be rejected in whole or in part, or (3) more information is required for a determination.

Such information can also be used for analysis, notably to assess, report, and improve quality. Health care providers could use the information to measure trends in their industry and assess the complex relationships among patient conditions, treatments, and outcomes. The results of this analysis might suggest alternative protocols or inform providers that they should specialize in certain cases and not others. Payers may be able to assess the quality and efficiency of providers and post such information publicly or use it to guide those they insure toward more cost-effective treatment centers. They could also use it to negotiate costs and premiums. The public health community could analyze information to draw conclusions over the entire universe of health care interventions. Analysis of codes can be used not only to adjust rates in general but to help clients get the most effective (or at least the most cost-effective) treatment for their conditions by identifying patients for disease management programs. How effectively codes are in fact used for purposes in which they could be used is another matter.

How the Codes Would Change

Understanding the impact of changing from ICD-9 to ICD-10 requires understanding how the codes themselves have changed. This section makes several points:

- Both ICD-10-CM and ICD-10-PCS offer more granularity and permit finer distinctions than do their predecessors. In addition, ICD-10-CM drops some distinctions no longer deemed relevant.
- Both ICD-10-CM and ICD-10-PCS have a different encoding format than their predecessors.
- ICD-10-PCS is almost a complete one-to-many expansion of ICD-9-CM, Volume 3: Almost every ICD-10-PCS code maps back into one and only one ICD-9-CM, Volume 3 code. ICD-10-CM, however, is an incomplete one-to-many expansion of ICD-9-CM, Volumes 1 and 2. In some cases, the distinctions may be better; however, the mapping from the new back into the old can be complex, as the next susbsection explains.
- ICD-10-CM is an evolution from its predecessor. ICD-10-PCS is a radical departure from the past.

The development of ICD-10-CM and ICD-10-PCS has proceeded along two completely different paths. In many ways, they have nothing in common but their name.

ICD-10-CM

When WHO issued ICD-9, U.S. health officials, increasingly interested in having these codes support health reporting and billing, concluded that they were incomplete without clinical modifications. These modifications—ICD-9-CM, Volumes 1 and 2—increased the number of codes by over half.

Fifteen years later, WHO developed ICD-10, which reflected advances in scientific and clinical knowledge over the prior 15 years and also included many—but by no means all—of the modifications made in the United States to ICD-9 that transformed it into ICD-9-CM, Volumes 1 and 2. In creating ICD-10-CM, therefore, CDC revisited the parts of ICD-9-CM that did not make it into ICD-10 and fit them into the new structure of ICD-10.

In the meantime, advances in understanding that could not wait for wholesale code revisions were incorporated into the annual updates of ICD-9-CM, Volumes 1 and 2. Roughly 1 percent of all codes are additions to or modifications of those from the year before. Even as ICD-10-CM is being weighed for adoption, ICD-9-CM continues to evolve, but not necessarily enough to accommodate every single advance in medical knowledge.

ICD-9-CM is mostly[3] a series of four-digit and some five-digit codes rendered as "XXX.X" or "XXX.XX" for diagnoses and as "XX.XX" for procedures. The first character in an ICD-10 code is a letter rather than a digit. ICD-10-CM differs further in having, alternatively, one, two, and (mostly to make left-right distinctions) three characters (numbers) after

---

[3] ICD-9-CM also contains "E" and "V" codes that describe the source of some diagnoses; these start with the letters "E" or "V".

the decimal point[4] (plus in some cases a fourth character to indicate whether the condition was encountered previously). Its field size is thus longer, which has ramifications for existing, albeit inflexible, computer systems.

In 1997, a crosswalk was developed between ICD-9-CM and ICD-10-CM (see the last section of this appendix for a discussion of crosswalks). The key issue in any such crosswalk, apart from its accuracy, is whether any given code maps back into one and only one old code (because new codes have greater specificity, many old codes map into multiple new codes). A new code that is a uniform many-to-one expansion of an old code is generally far easier to switch to than one that is not. New codes can be dealt with by being mapped into old codes and processed the same way old codes were. Many payers, for instance, use an elaborate decision logic to determine whether or how much to pay on a claim; such logic is often based on the diagnostic and procedure codes submitted. If a new code is a one-to-one expansion of the old code, then it is possible for payers to translate every new code into an old code, make determinations based on the old code, and then pick up the new code again once the calculations are made. Payers may, at their later discretion, choose to treat each of the many new codes (those that map into one old code) differently. Presumably, if they do, it is only because it is in their interest to do so (i.e., it is not a net cost). In contrast, whenever a new code maps to more than one old code, it is unclear which of the old codes provides the logic that applies to the new code.

According to the 1997 crosswalk, 12,566 ICD-9-CM codes[5] expanded to 19,019 ICD-10-CM codes, about a third of which were carried over directly from WHO's ICD-10 standard. The rest were more detailed clinical modifications of WHO's codes. Roughly 31,000 six-character codes—or almost 65,000 if seventh-character extensions are counted (a disproportionate share of which describe injuries)—are not specifically listed on the crosswalk. The various parts of the ICD-9 code expanded in uneven fashion. On average, for instance, there was only a slight expansion of codes for diseases (with the exception of tuberculosis; see below) and pregnancy/childbirth conditions. In contrast, there was a fivefold expansion in the number of codes for bones and muscles, and a fourfold expansion for injuries. When the latter two categories are omitted, the overall expansion ratio in the number of codes is 90 percent.

Overall, the changes made from ICD-9-CM to ICD-10-CM cannot be characterized simply. In infectious diseases alone, there is a good deal more detail (e.g., typhoid, diphtheria, Lyme disease) and there are many diseases for which certain qualifying details were dropped even as other details were added. The latter include polio (types 1, 2, and 3 polio were no longer coded as separate diseases), pneumonic plague (primary and secondary plague were no longer held to be distinct), and tuberculosis. Some of these changes originated in the switch from ICD-9 to ICD-10.

ICD-9-CM has 392 unique codes to describe tuberculosis in its many sites within the body and manifestations. ICD-10-CM has only 44 unique codes for tuberculosis. Ostensibly, detail is being lost. However, as an example, one type of tuberculosis, vertebral tuberculosis, is represented by one code in ICD-10-CM but by seven codes in ICD-9-CM. The ad-

---

[4] Many ICD codes—specifically, those for injuries—have a seventh character extension to provide further information. A common seventh character indicates whether the encounter is an "initial encounter," a "subsequent encounter," or a "sequela."

[5] As of October 2002, there were 12,924 codes.

ditional codes in ICD-9-CM indicate on which test the diagnosis is based (i.e., histological, cultural, micro, no examination, unknown examination, examination not elsewhere classified, and examination not otherwise stated). This pattern continues the entire way through the list of tuberculosis-related diagnoses. Since TB is now confirmed by PCR (polymerase chain reaction) identification of *M. tuberculosis,* discarding the now-meaningless information about tests leaves 50 unique ICD-9-CM codes in comparison with 44 unique ICD-10-CM codes. In some cases, correct diagnoses for tuberculosis requires two ICD-10-CM codes, whereas one ICD-9-CM code sufficed earlier.

The fact that one ICD-10-CM code can be mapped into multiple ICD-9-CM codes matters less if the distinctions among the older codes are of little relevance (e.g., older data that used either of the multiple ICD-9-CM codes could probably have been lumped together and nothing much would have been lost). That leaves the question of how widely people in the industry make choices (e.g., payment eligibility) based on distinctions now known to be meaningless. The realization that these distinctions, in retrospect, should never have been part of the claims logic might provide cold comfort to those who have to bear the cost of reprogramming their information systems to handle ICD-10-CM.

Once due account is taken of ICD-9-CM code distinctions that are no longer clinically meaningful (so that an arbitrary back-mapping into one of the old codes is acceptable), ICD-10-CM appears closer to being a one-to-many expansion of ICD-9-CM. The increase in its specificity is somewhat greater than the raw numbers indicate.

ICD-10-PCS

At the same time as ICD-9 was modified to generate ICD-9-CM, Volumes 1 and 2, ICD-9-CM, Volume 3, was also being developed. Despite its title, this code set was in no way derived from ICD-9; it was developed as a separate effort.

The development of ICD-10-PCS was prompted because ICD-9-CM, Volume 3, is simply running out of room. ICD-9-CM, Volume 3, codes are four numeric digits long—large enough to express a space of 10,000 possibilities, of which 3,500 are designated codes. Although the code space was not absolutely exhausted, many of the two-digit categories were. For instance, the code space (37.xx) for cardiology procedures is effectively full; code designers must find more codes in previously unused parts of the code space (e.g., 00.xx) for new procedures, which permitted a handful of new procedures to be coded. However, it meant that people looking for cardiac procedures had to look both in expected places (37.xx) and elsewhere (00.xx).

Assigning new procedure codes randomly would mean that the problem of code-space exhaustion could be postponed for a long time. Computer lookup tables could be used to map codes into broader categories; one could then search on the broader categories (e.g., all cardiology procedures). Doing so would permit such information to be recovered but would call for a major readjustment in analytic techniques (e.g., one could not simply search on the first two digits of a code alone); such reprogramming is not cost-free.[6] It would also put an end to the practice of glancing at a code and knowing what category it referred to, since the codes themselves would have as much meaning as the last four digits of U.S. phone numbers do.

---

[6]Adjustments would also have to be made to legacy systems that access data stores sequentially (and that store procedure records in numeric order rather than randomly).

The difficulties of finding new code space have led to a reluctance to assign new codes to new procedures unless the requirement was felt to be particularly urgent. New codes have been found for about a dozen of the more common laparoscopies (e.g., appendix removal and colostomy), but far more of the laparoscopy procedures have been lumped with open surgery procedures. Those who want to look at hospital discharge records to determine whether laparoscopies were effective (e.g., Did patients have to return more often for further treatment?) would be frustrated by the difficulty of differentiating between laparoscopies and open surgery procedures in any but the few more commonly performed procedures. Other new procedures (such as interventional radiology) were also lumped in with older, more general procedural codes.

ICD-10-PCS was created for CMS from the ground up between 1995 and 1998 by 3M Health Information Systems. It was based on an analysis of Medicare Provider Analysis and Review (MEDPAR) files, consistent with principles laid out by NCVHS in the early 1990s. The first five of those principles specified that the code be

- *comprehensive:* all procedures are classified
- *unique:* all substantially different procedures have a unique code
- *expandable:* new procedures can be incorporated as new codes
- *hierarchical:* individual codes are aggregated into larger categories
- *standardized:* all terminology is precisely defined.

These criteria are not unusual. All code sets should adhere, at least nominally, to these principles—and most do. The next two criteria gave ICD-10-PCS its defining features. The code should also be

- *strictly procedural:* procedure descriptions contain no diagnostic information
- *multi-axial:* each code character has a consistent meaning.

The result was a code that was long (7 characters), capacious (52 billion theoretical combinations), and multi-axial.[7] The multi-axial coding scheme has some advantages; one can look at a code and guess what it means without knowing its definition. The 30 root operations[8] coded by the third alphanumeric are the same regardless of what part of the body is under discussion. Anyone who memorizes the small set of words that represent body system and root operations will know what the first three characters of the medical/surgical codes

---

[7] *Multi-axial* means that each of the seven alphanumeric characters stands for something specific within every section (although the meaning of the code shifts differs within each of the major sections, the shift is modest), regardless of which subcategory of code it belongs to. In other words, the hierarchical declension is invariant within every section. The first character refers to the broad procedure category, of which "medical and surgical" is likely to get the most attention among the 16 sections of the standard (it accounts for over 90 percent of the codes). Each code of the medical and surgical section starts with "0". The next six characters in that section (and the obstetrics section) are assigned as follows: The second character refers to the body system; the third, to the root operation; the fourth, to the body part or region; the fifth, to the approach (how the procedure is done: e.g., open surgery, percutaneous, etc.); the sixth, to a device left in the patient (may also refer to, e.g., blood transfusions); and the seventh, to all qualifiers. For more detail See Richard F. Averill et al., "Development of the ICD-10 Procedure Coding System (ICD-10-PCS)," 3M Health Information System Research Report, April 1998.

[8] Alteration, bypass, change, control, creation, destruction, detachment, dilation, division, drainage, excision, extirpation, extraction, fragmentation, fusion, insertion, inspection, map, occlusion, reattachment, release, removal, repair, replacement, reposition, resection, restriction, revision, transfer, and transplantation.

refer to without having to memorize 200,000 cases. To a lesser extent, similar ease of use (not having to look things up) also characterizes the next three axes.

But the advantages are not free. In most codes, the early characters contain the more important distinctions; the later characters contain finer distinctions. In ICD-10-PCS, the key distinctions may be in the fourth, fifth, or sixth characters. Some procedures may best be differentiated in ways other than what any of the seven fixed axes clearly expresses. Although the 34-character alphanumeric set makes it highly unlikely that the number of distinct differentiations along any axis will exceed what the code allows, it also leads to codes that are hard to memorize. Overall, the code space of ICD-10-PCS is sparsely but not evenly populated.

One particularly noteworthy feature of ICD-10-PCS is its relative reduction of NOS and NEC codes,[9] which forces caregivers and coders to be specific about the kind of procedures used[10] (and which may therefore require that more work be put into coding). ICD-9, in contrast, is replete with such codes. The heavy use of such codes makes it difficult to see the detail in the data. In reviewing spinal surgeries (the more specific types of which postdate the drafting of ICD-9-CM), Dr. Tom Faciszewski et al., describing 143 operative interventions, found that 46 percent of the ICD codes included the NEC designation, leaving only 164 assigned ICD codes compared with 428 specific CPT codes assigned for the same spine procedures.[11] The result is that ICD-9-CM procedure coding may lack detail and may misidentify spine surgical procedures.

ICD-10-PCS specifically avoids compound procedure sets. However, software can be written that automatically translates common compound procedures into a series of ICD-10-PCS primitives (similar to the constituent words that make up compound words).[12]

ICD-10-PCS also records many procedures as taking place along the "upper," "middle," or "lower" as well as to the "greater" or "lesser" part of an organ or circulation system. If errors are not to be added, such details would have to become standard in patient records.

---

[9] Many codes in ICD-10-CM are of the form Condition X NEC, and Condition X NOS. When NEC or NOS is used, a subcategorization is generally implied. That is, one may have codes as follows: Condition X subcategory A, Condition X subcategory B, Condition X subcategory C, Condition X NEC, and Condition X NOS. Here, NEC means that the diagnosis is known to be condition X but also known not to fall into either subcategory A, subcategory B, or subcategory C. NOS means that the subcategory is unknown. For NEC to make sense, one must know the existence of subcategories A, B, and C. Obviously, if one adds a category D the next year, then the definition of Condition X NEC will also change —something that must be factored in when making year-to-year comparisons. For NOS to make sense, one must know that subcategories exist at all. Within a code arranged in (alpha-) numeric order, this is straightforward. If one uses words, these distinctions may not be so clear. The words themselves must be arranged carefully and there must be no cases where Condition X subcategory A is known in the profession by other words entirely. All this can be expressed through lookup tables unless it is considered undesirable that lookup tables be part of the standard itself.

[10] The head of ICD-10-PCS's development team, Richard Averill, illustrated the 48 codes applicable for dilation of the heart and great vessels, giving three choices for the device inserted: intraluminal device, device NEC, and none. Note that the coder is not allowed to disregard the issue of whether a device was or was not left in the body—i.e., device NOS is not a legitimate code. The choice is between a specific device, some other device, and no device. So the coder must determine (1) whether a device was or was not left in, and (2) whether the device was or was not an intraluminal device.

[11] Tom Faciszewski et al., "Procedural Coding of Spinal Surgeries (CPT-4 versus ICD-9-CM) and Decisions Regarding Standards: a Multicenter Study" *Spine,* Vol. 28, No. 5, 2003, pp. 502–507.

[12] What in ICD-9-CM, Volume 3, for instance, is a bilateral Salpingo-Oophorectomy (65.61), in ICD-10-PCS is broken down into a Salpingectomy (0VR60ZZ) and an Oophorectom (OVR20ZZ). This broad rule has plusses and minuses, among them that familiar procedures (e.g., a Whipple procedure) have no obvious code in ICD-10-PCS. This means that there is no obvious way to state that a set of sequential procedures is, in fact, one overall procedure and should be billed at that rate. Nevertheless, such an objection should be put into perspective. Defenders of ICD-10-PCS also retort that the Whipple procedure does not have a unique definition; it varies from practice to practice. Also, software that allows user-defined entries can permit such differences to be accommodated correctly.

Above all, ICD-10-PCS is a radical change in the number of codes: from 3,500 in ICD-9-CM, Volume 3, to almost 200,000[13] codes (plus radiology codes[14]). Such a large code size virtually guarantees that ICD-10-PCS *is* almost entirely a one-to-many expansion of its predecessor.[15] Fewer than 100 old codes map to two new codes, but no old code maps to more than two. Conversely, in many cases, hundreds or even thousands of new codes would replace one old code. Indeed, 27 ICD-9-CM, Volume 3, codes map into more than a thousand ICD-10-PCS codes. Code 39.49 (other revision of vascular procedure) has been replaced by 19,217 new ICD-10-PCS codes; code 34.99—other operations on the thorax—has been expanded to 8,033 new codes.

The Importance of Crosswalks and Mappings

One of the most important considerations in reducing the costs and enhancing the benefits of moving from ICD-9 to ICD-10 is the quality of the mapping from one to the other. Good mappings, which are largely a characteristic of the code definitions themselves, ease the cost of transition by permitting the logic that is used for old codes (e.g., to determine whether the medical care given is covered by insurance) to be carried over to the new ones. It also permits old data to be meaningfully combined with new data to create a time series that smoothly spans the transition between code sets.

Mappings between codes are the logical consequence of mappings between conditions in the real world and their rendering as codes. To illustrate this, imagine a set consisting of all possible diagnoses of a particular type. Each diagnosis is mapped into a diagnostic code in ICD-9-CM and mapped again into a diagnostic code in ICD-10-CM.

The two codes can be said to be in *one-to-one mapping* if every diagnosis that was associated with one ICD-9-CM code is associated with only one ICD-10-CM code. This is illustrated by Figure A.2, which, like the next three figures, classifies eight sample diagnoses *a* through *h* (note that the codes used are not real; they are made-up examples). In this case, the transition from one code to another is easy: Wherever one ICD-9-CM name comes up in the database or code logic, it can be replaced with a corresponding ICD-10-CM name. All time series continue smoothly.

---

[13] This and subsequent data come from a crosswalk developed between ICD-10-PCS and ICD-9-CM, Volume 3, and may, for that reason, present statistics that differ from other sources.

[14] The nine old radiology codes of ICD-9-CM, Volume 3, would be replaced by more than 60,000 codes in ICD-10-PCS. CMS, however, does not use radiology codes to determine DRGs.

[15] Diagnoses tell what Mother Nature did to the patient and can be reinterpreted in the light of later science. Thus, code hierarchies may be later found to be misleading. In contrast, procedures tell what people do; they are what they are and would very rarely be reinterpreted in the light of later science. In the latter case, hierarchies of procedures are more likely to be stable in the light of new science.

Figure A.2
An Example of One-to-One Mapping

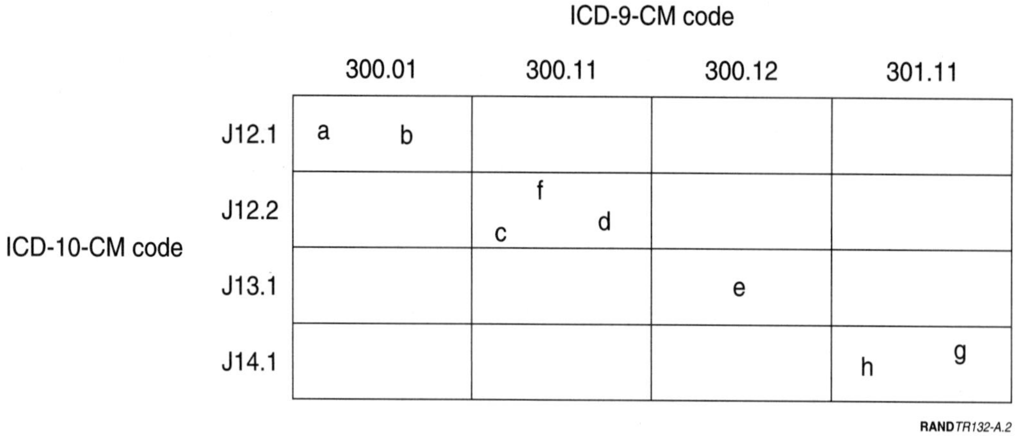

	ICD-9-CM code			
ICD-10-CM code	300.01	300.11	300.12	301.11
J12.1	a b			
J12.2		f c d		
J13.1			e	
J14.1				h g

RAND*TR132-A.2*

In Figure A.3, the four categories of ICD-9-CM map into the six categories of ICD-10-CM. This is a clean *one-to-many* expansion, which increases the amount of information provided. Diagnosis *c* is differentiated from diagnoses *f* and *d* (and similarly for diagnoses *g* and *h*). Here, one can construct a consistent time series by mapping everything *back* into ICD-9-CM (one loses the new distinctions that the newer codes embody, but such information was never collected under the old code). Payers that have devised medical-necessity judgments based on diagnoses under the old code could, at least initially, have an easier transition by translating the new diagnostic codes into the old diagnostic codes, and applying the logic that applied to the old code.

Figure A.3
A Clean One-to-Many Expansion Increases the Amount of Information Provided

	ICD-9-CM code			
ICD-10-CM code	300.01	300.11	300.12	301.11
J12.1	a b			
J12.2		c		
J13.1			e	
J13.2				h
J13.3		f d		
J14.1				g

RAND*TR132-A.3*

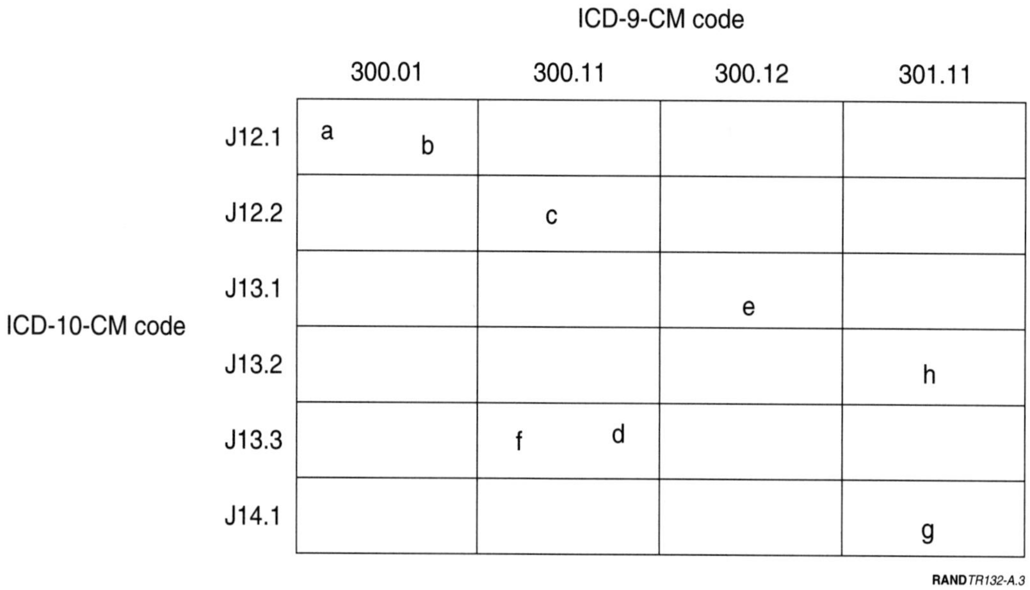

Figure A.4 shows the reverse; the four categories of ICD-9-CM map into the three categories of ICD-10-CM. This is a clean *many-to-one* contraction, in which information is lost. Diagnosis *e*, which once merited treatment separate from diagnoses *g* and *h*, is now coded the same way (but perhaps the information lost was later deemed to be a distinction without a difference). One can still construct a good time series by mapping everything *forward* into ICD-10-CM, but distinctions that were present in the old data would be lost (again, perhaps deservedly). The change creates a problem for payers, particularly those that treated diagnosis *e* differently (as 300.12) than diagnoses *g* and *h* (as 301.11). They must decide whether to treat *e, g,* and *h* as they would have treated *e* or as they would have treated *g* and *h*. The option to treat them separately no longer exists (the payer has no way of knowing from discharge data whether something encoded as J13.1 was diagnosis *e, g,* or *h*).

Figure A.4
The Reverse of Figure A.3: In a Many-to-One Contraction, Information Is Lost

		ICD-9-CM code			
		300.01	300.11	300.12	301.11
ICD-10-CM code	J12.1	a b			
	J12.2		c d f		
	J13.1			e	g h

RAND *TR132-A.4*

Figure A.5 on the next page illustrates a *many-to-many* mapping. Even though the new codes may be more accurate ways to group diagnoses, it is no longer easy to construct reliable time series or to use the old logic to treat the new codes. There is no way of knowing whether a condition with a new code of J12.1 was diagnosis *a* (and thus would have been 300.01) or diagnosis *f* (and thus would have been 300.11). Thus, the only way to construct an accurate time series (short of looking at every medical record) is to create super-categories, lumping together cases coded as 300.01 and 300.11, and those coded as J12.1 and J12.2. Information is lost in both directions. Similarly, if payers treat 300.01 and 300.11 cases differently, they will have to revisit and revise their logic altogether when they get cases coded as J12.1 or J12.2.

Figure A.5
A Many-to-Many Mapping

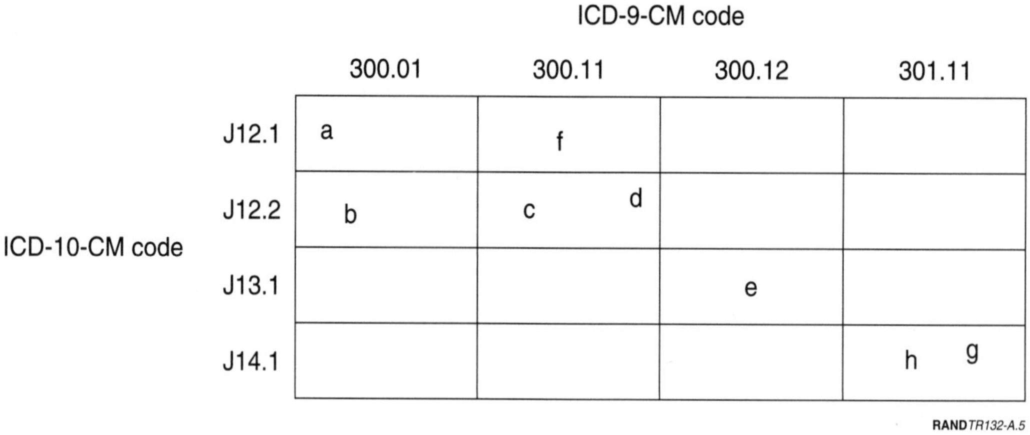

ICD-9-CM code

	300.01	300.11	300.12	301.11
J12.1	a	f		
J12.2	b	c d		
J13.1			e	
J14.1				h g

ICD-10-CM code

List of Interviewees

(All interviews were conducted in 2003.)

Experts: George Goldberg, independent consultant (April 14); Lee Hillborne, RAND (April 14); Chris Chute, Mayo Foundation (April 18); Bart McCann, Health Policy Alternatives (May 13); Lisa Iezzoni, Harvard Medical School (May 14); Cheryl Damberg, RAND (May 22); Prinny Rose Abraham, National Association of Home Care (May 28); Eric Schneider, Harvard Medical School (June 2); Arnie Millstein, Pacific Business Group on Health (July 7); Elaine Power, National Quality Forum (July 8); Jim Cimino, Columbia University (July 17); Marge Zernott, ZKC Associates (July 21); Edward Sondik, NCHS (July 24); Vergil Slee, Tringa Group (July 29); Patrick Romano, University of California at Davis (July 31); David Classen, First Consulting Group (August 4); Mayer Davidson, Drew University (August 13).

Associations: Sue Prophet-Bowman and Dan Rode, AHIMA (10 April); Nelly Leon-Chisen, AHA (April 17); Michael Beebe, Jack Emery, Cornwell Smith, and Pam Curlin, American Medical Association (April 22); Teresa Doyle and Bill Alfano, Blue Cross Blue Shield Association (May 12); Richard Landen, Blue Cross Blue Shield Association (May 2); Tom Musco and Michael DeCarlo, Health Insurance Association of America (May 13); Lenore Whalen, Federation of American Hospitals (May 15); Melissa Bartlett, American Association of Health Plans (May 29); Joyce Sensmeier, Healthcare Information and Management Systems Society (July 8); Carol Bickford, American Nursing Association (July 9); Denise Love, National Association of Health Data Organizations (July 31); Margaret VanAmringe, Joint Commission on Accreditation of Healthcare Organizations (July 31).

Providers: Elaine Schneider, Greater Baltimore Medical Center (April 23); Sue Tierney and Judy Krohn, Marshfield Clinic (May 20); Doug Wood, Mayo Clinic (May 27); Blackford Middleton, Partners HealthCare (May 29); Kathy Anderson, Greater Baltimore Medical Center (June 2); Cathy Colton, Harvard Pilgrim (June 13); Mike Fedor, Kaiser Permanente (June 25); Andy Wiesenthal, Kaiser Permanente (June 25); Gil Kuperman, Partners HealthCare (July 14); Gail Garrett, HCA (July 18); Karen Rutledge, Tenet Healthcare Corporation (July 21); Greg Walton, Carilion Health (July 22); Janie Cilo, Craig Hospital (July 22); Diana Stump, Northwest Community Hospital (July 25); Mark Sell, Aurora Health Care (July 28); Judy Snipes, Carilion Health System (July 30); Pam Wirth, Susquehanna Health (July 31); David Bates, Brigham and Women's Hospital (August 4).

Payers: Jim Daley, Blue Cross and Blue Shield of South Carolina (May 14 and 27); Nancy Engel, United Healthcare (May 28); James Cross, Aetna (May 29); Chris Apkar, Providence Health (June 5); Claudia Melendrez, Presbyterian (June 11); Robert Perlitz, Empire Blue Cross Blue Shield (June 13); Jack McCrae, Mike Heuer, and Dr. Castiglia,

Premera Blue Cross (June 20); Jim Coan, Aetna (June 23); Dennis Angeles, Presbyterian (July 18).

Software and Service Vendors: Richard Averill, 3M Health Information Services (April 17 and July 29); Louise Smith, Ellen Arnold, and Gerald McAllister, McKesson (June 19); Sheri Bernard, Ingenix (July 7); Susan deCathelineau, QuadraMed (July 11); Ian Chuang, Cerner (July 15); Kim Stafford, Solucient (July 16); Darryl Landis, CorSolutions (July 18); Russell Robbins, Symmetry (July 21); Karen White, Medstat (July 22).

Government (United States, Canada, and Australia): Rosemary Roberts, National Centre for Classification in Health, Australia (e-mail, May 29); Robert Davis, State of New York (April 21); Lori Moskal and Diana Calfield, Canadian Institute for Health Information (May 13); Yen Pin Chiang, AHRQ (May 20); Patricia Brooks, CMS (May 22); Bill Baine, AHRQ (May 23); Karen Trudel, CMS (May 28); Betsy Humphries, National Library of Medicine (June 3); Gail Graham, Veterans Administration (June 20); Yolanda Robinson, CMS (July 9); Michael Fitzmaurice, AHRQ (July 11); Helen Whittome, Ontario Ministry of Health and Long-Term Care (July 11); Tom Gustafson, CMS (July 16); Janet Kramer, Office of the Inspector General, Department of Health and Human Services (July 22); Julie Wolcott, Institute of Medicine (July 29); Marvin Ross, Illinois Department of Public Assistance (July 30).

Bibliography

Abraham, Prinny Rose, "ICD-9 Raises Concerns for Home Health Information Managers," *Journal of AHIMA*, Vol. 73, No. 5, May 2002, pp. 62–64.

Aspen Systems Corporation, *Issues Related to the Use of ICD-10-PCS as the Single Procedure Code Set*, Prepared for the American Medical Association, May 1999.

Averill, Richard A., Robert Mullin, Barbara Steinbeck, Norbert Goldfield, and Thelma Grant, *Development of the ICD-10 Procedure Coding System (ICD-10-PCS)*, 3M HIS Research Report, April 1998.

Benesch, C., D. M. Witter, Jr., A. L. Wilder, P. W. Duncan, G. P. Samsa, and D. B. Matchar, "Inaccuracy of the International Classification of Diseases (ICD-9-CM) in Identifying the Diagnosis of Ischemic Cerebrovascular Disease," *Neurology*, Vol. 49, No. 3, September 1997, pp. 660–664.

Berthelsen, Cheryl, "Evaluation of Coding Data Quality of the HCUP National Inpatient Sample," *Topics in Health Information Management*, Vol. 21, No. 2, 2000, pp. 10–23.

Boyles, Sarah Hamilton, Anne Weber, and Leslie Meyn, "Procedures for Pelvic Organ Prolapse in the United States, 1979-1997," *American Journal of Obstetrics and Gynecology*, Vol. 188, No. 1, January 2003, pp. 108–115.

Brooks, Patricia E., "Testing ICD-10-PCS," *Journal of AHIMA*, Vol. 69, No. 5, May 1998, pp. 73–74.

Carter, Grace, M., and Paul B. Ginsburg, *The Medicare Case Mix Index Increase: Medical Practice Changes, Aging, and DRG Creep*, Santa Monica, Calif.: RAND, R-3292-HCFA, 1985.

Centers for Medicare and Medicaid Services, "Health Care Industry Market Update, Acute Care Hospitals," July 14, 2003, cms.hhs.gov/reports/hcimu/hcimu_07142003.pdf.

Chaiken, Barry P., and Donald Holmquest, "Patient Safety: Modifying Processes to Eliminate Medical Errors," *Journal of Quality Health Care*, Vol. 1, No. 2, April/June 2002, pp. 20–23.

Cimino, J. J., "Saying What You Mean and Meaning What You Say: Coupling Biomedical Terminology and Knowledge," *Academic Medicine*, Vol. 68, No. 4, April 1993, pp. 257–260.

Cimino, J. J., "Review Paper: Coding Systems in Health Care," *Methods of Information in Medicine*, No. 35, 1996, pp. 273–284.

Cimino, J. J., "Desiderata for Controlled Medical Vocabularies in the Twenty-First Century," *Methods of Information in Medicine*, No. 37, 1998, pp. 394–403.

Connecting for Health: A Public-Private Collaborative, The Data Standards Working Group, Markle Foundation, June 5, 2003.

Coopers & Lybrand, *Cost-Benefit Analysis of a Uniform Procedural Coding System for Physician Services*, Report prepared for the American Medical Association, Chicago, IL, September 1989.

"The Cost of SARS: $11 Billion and Rising," *Far Eastern Economic Review*, Vol. 166, No.16, 2003, p. 12.

Derby, Carol A., Kate L. Lapane, Henry A. Feldman, and Richard A. Carleton, "Possible Effect of DRGs on the Classification of Stroke: Implications for Epidemiological Surveillance," *Stroke: Journal of the American Heart Association*, Vol. 32, No. 7, July 2001, pp.1487–1491.

Dimitropoulos, Vera, "The Introduction of ICD-10-AM in Health Information Management Education at the University of Sydney," *Health Information Management,* Vol. 28, No. 2, 1998, pp. 88–92.

Faciszewski, Tom, Steven K. Broste, and David Fardon, "Quality of Data Regarding Diagnoses of Spinal Disorders in Administrative Databases: A Multicenter Study," *The Journal of Bone and Joint Surgery*, Vol. 79-A, No. 10, October 1997, pp. 1481–1488.

Faciszewski, Tom, Ron Jensen, and Richard L. Berg, "Procedural Coding of Spinal Surgeries (CPT-4 versus ICD-9-CM) and Decisions Regarding Standards: A Multicenter Study," *Spine*, Vol. 28, No. 5, March 1, 2003, pp. 502–507.

Fintor, Lou, "Health Agencies Adopt New Disease Classification Codes," *Journal of the National Cancer Institute,* No. 94, May 15, 2002, pp. 710–711.

Fisher, E. S., F. S. Whaley, W. M. Krushat, D. J. Malenka, C. Fleming, J. A. Baron, D. C. Hsia, "The Accuracy of Medicare's Hospital Claims Data: Progress Has Been Made, but Problems Remain," *American Journal of Public Health*, Vol. 82, No. 2, February, 1992, pp. 243–248.

Fishman, Paul A., Michael J. Goodman, Mark C. Hornbrook, Richard Meenan, Donal Bachman, and Maureen C. O'Keefe Rosetti, "Risk-Adjustment Using Automated Ambulatory Pharmacy Data: The RxRisk Model," *Medical Care*, Vol. 41, No. 1, January 2003, pp. 84–99.

Fishman, Paul A. and David Shay, "Development and Estimation of a Pediatric Chronic Disease Score Using Automated Pharmacy Data," *Medical Care*, Vol. 37, No. 9, September 1999, pp. 874–883.

General Accounting Office (GAO), "Federal Budget, Opportunities for Oversight and Improved Use of Taxpayer Funds," Statement of David M. Walker, Comptroller General of the United States, Washington, D.C.: GAO-03-922T, June 2003.

_____, *HIPPA Standards: Dual Code Sets Are Acceptable for Reporting Medical Procedures*, Washington, D.C.: GAO-02-796, August 2002.

Geraci, Jane M., "The Demise of Comparative Provider Complication Rates Derived from ICD-9-CM Code Diagnoses," *Medical Care*, Vol. 40, No. 10, October 2002, pp. 847–850.

Geraci, Jane M., Carol M. Ashton, David H. Kuykendall, Michael L. Johnson, and Louis Wu, "International Classification of Diseases, 9th Revision, Clinical Modification Codes in Discharge Abstracts Are Poor Measures of Complication Occurrence in Medical Inpatients," *Medical Care*, Vol. 35, No. 6, June 1997, pp. 589–602.

Gillespie, Greg, "Shining Light into the Depths of Databases," *Health Data Management*, April 29, 2003, http://www.healthdatamanagement.com/HDMSearchResultsDetails.cfm?DID=13081.

Goldstein, Larry B., "Accuracy of ICD-9-CM Coding for the Identification of Patients with Acute Ischemic Stroke: Effect of Modifier Codes, *Stroke: A Journal of Cerebral Circulation*, Vol. 29, No. 8, August 1998, pp. 1602–1604.

Grigg, Betty, et al., "Coding Changes and Apparent HIV/AIDS Mortality Trends in Florida, 1999," *Journal of the American Medical Association,* Vol. 286, No. 15, 2001, p. 1839.

Guevara, Ramon, Jay C. Butler, Barbara Marston, and Joseph Plouffe, "Accuracy of ICD-9-CM Codes in Detecting Community-Acquired Pneumococcal Pneumonia for Incidence and Vaccine Efficacy Studies," *American Journal of Epidemiology*, Vol. 149, No. 3, February 1, 1999, pp. 282–289.

Hall, Keri K., John Philbrick, and Mohan Nadkarni, "Evaluation and Treatment of Acute Bronchitis at an Academic Teaching Clinic," *The American Journal of the Medical Sciences*, Vol. 325, No. 1, January 2003, pp. 7–9.

Hazlet, Thomas K., Todd A. Lee, Philip D. Hansten, and John R. Horn, "Performance of Community Pharmacy Drug Interaction Software," *Journal of the American Pharmaceutical Association*, Vol. 41, No. 2, 2001, pp. 200–204.

Hebden, Joan, and Mary-Claire Roghmann, "Use of ICD-9-CM Coding as a Case-Finding Method for Sternal Wound Infections after CABG Procedures," *American Journal of Infection Control*, Vol. 28, No. 2, April 2000, pp. 202–203.

Hornbrook, Mark C., Michael J. Goodman, Paul A. Fishman, Richard T. Meenan, Maureen O'Keefe-Rosetti, and Donald J. Bachman, "Building Health Plan Databases to Risk Adjust Outcomes and Payments," *International Journal for Quality in Health Care*, Vol. 10, No. 6, 1998, pp. 531–538.

Iezzoni, Lisa I., ed., *Risk Adjustment for Measuring Health Care Outcomes*, Ann Arbor, MI: Health Administration Press, 1994.

Iezzoni, Lisa I., "Assessing Quality Using Administrative Data," *Annals of Internal Medicine*, Vol. 127, 1997, pp. 666–674.

Innes, Kerry, Karen Peasley, and Rosemary Roberts, "Ten Down Under: Implementing ICD-10 in Australia," *Journal of AHIMA*, Vol. 71, No. 1, January 2000, pp. 52–56.

Kloss, Linda, "ICD-10: Regulations May Be on the Way," *Journal of AHIMA*, Vol. 73, No. 7, July–August 2002, p. 29.

Lawthers, E., Heather R. Palmer, and Lisa Iezzoni, "Identification of In-Hospital Complications from Claims Data: Is It Valid?" *Medical Care*, Vol. 38, No. 8, August 2000, pp. 785–795.

LeMier, M., P. Cummings, and T. A. West, "Accuracy of External Cause of Injury Codes Reported in Washington State Hospital Discharge Records," *Injury Prevention*, No. 7, 2001, pp. 334–338.

Lesar, Timothy, "Recommendations for Reducing Medication Errors," *Medscape Pharmacists*, Vol. 1, No. 2, 2000, http://www.medscape.com/viewarticle/408566.

Lewis, Michael D., Julie A. Pavlin, Jay L. Mansfield, Sheilah O'Brien, Louis G. Boomsma, Yevgeniy Elbert, and Patrick W. Kelley, "Disease Outbreak Detection System Using Syndromic Data in the Greater Washington DC Area," *American Journal of Preventive Medicine*, Vol. 23, No. 3, 2002, pp. 180–186.

Mayo, Robert R., and Richard D. Swartz, "Redefining the Incidence of Clinically Detectable Atheroembolism," *American Journal of Medicine*, Vol. 100, No. 5, May 1996, pp. 524–529.

McGlynn, Elizabeth, "An Evidence-Based Quality Measurement and Reporting System," *Medical Care*, Vol. 41, No.1, Supplement, 2003, pp. I-8–I-15.

Moving Toward International Standards in Primary Care Information: Clinical Vocabulary, AHRQ & AMIA Conference Summary Report, New Orleans, LA, November 1995.

Muldoon, John H., "Structure and Performance of Different DRG Classification Systems for Neonatal Medicine," *Pediatrics*, Vol. 103, No. 1, January 1999, pp. 302–318.

National Centre for Classification in Health, "Comparison of ICD-9-CM and ICD-10-AM," *Health Information Management*, Vol. 27, No. 1, 1997, pp. 23–27.

National Center for Health Statistics, *Ambulatory and Inpatient Procedures in the United States 1996*, November 1998.

_____, *2001 National Hospital Discharge Survey*, www.cdc.gov/nchs/about/major/hdasd/nhds.htm.

"New Classification for Deaths and Injuries Involving Terrorism," *Morbidity & Mortality Weekly Report*, Vol. 51, No. 36, 2002, pp. 18–19.

Ollendorf, Daniel, A. Mark Fendrick, Karen Massey, G. Rhys Williams, and Gerry Oster, "Is Sepsis Accurately Coded on Hospital Bills?" *Value in Health*, Vol. 5, No. 2, 2002, pp. 79–81.

Peden, Ann H., "An Overview of Coding and Its Relationship to Standardized Clinical Terminology," *Topics in Health Information Management*, Vol. 21, No. 2, 2000, pp. 1–9.

Petersen, Laura A., Steven Wright, Sharon-Lise Normand, and Jennifer Daley, "Positive Predictive Value of the Diagnosis of Acute Myocardial Infarction in an Administrative Database," *Journal of General Internal Medicine*," Vol. 14, No. 9, September 1999, pp. 555–558.

Piriyawat, Paisithl, Miriam Smajsova, Melinda Smith, Sanjay Pallegar, Areej Al-Wabil, Nelda Garcia, Jan Risser, Lemuel Moye, and Lewis Morgenstern, "Comparison of Active and Passive Surveillance for Cerebrovascular Disease: The Brain Attack Surveillance in Corpus Christi (BASIC) Project," *American Journal of Epidemiology*, Vol. 156, No. 11, December 1, 2002, pp. 1062–1069.

Prophet, Sue, "Testimony of the American Health Information Management Association to the National Committee on Vital and Health Statistics on ICD-10-CM," May 29, 2002.

Prophet, Sue, "ICD-10 on the Horizon," *Journal of AHIMA,* Vol. 73, No. 7, July–August 2002, pp. 36–41.

Reker, Dean M., Amy K. Rosen, Helen Hoenig, Dan Berlowitz, Judith Laughlin, Leigh Anderson, Clifford R. Marshall, and Maude Rittman, "The Hazards of Stroke Case Selection Using Administrative Data," *Medical Care*, Vol. 40, No. 2, February 2002, pp. 96–104.

Roberts, Rosemary F., Kerry C. Innes, and Susan M. Walker, "Introducing ICD-10-AM in Australian Hospitals," *Medical Journal of Australia*, Vol. 169, Supplement, October 19, 1998, pp. S32–S35.

Rode, Dan, "AHIMA Testifies in Support of ICD-10," *Journal of AHIMA,* Vol. 72, No. 7, July–August 2001, pp. 16–18.

Rode, Dan, "Taking Our Stand: AHIMA Stakes Four Key Issues," *Journal of AHIMA,* Vol. 73, No. 7, July–August 2002, pp. 24–26.

Romano, Patrick S., Benjamin K. Chan, Michael E. Schembri, and Julie A. Rainwater, "Can Administrative Data Be Used to Compare Postoperative Complication Rates Across Hospitals?" *Medical Care*, Vol. 40, No. 10, October 2002, pp. 856–867.

Romano, Patrick S., and Harold S. Luft, "Getting the Most Out of Messy Data: Problems and Approaches for Dealing with Large Administrative Data Sets," in *Summary Report: Medical Effectiveness Research Data Methods*, AHCPR Pub. No. 92-0056, July 1992, pp. 57–75.

Rosen, Amy, Jeanne Wu, Bei-Hung Chang, Dan Berlowitz, Arlene Ash, and Mark Moskowitz, "Does Diagnostic Information Contribute to Predicting Functional Decline in Long-Term Care?," *Medical Care*, Vol. 38, No. 6, June 2000, pp. 647–659.

Rudman, William J. and Calvin R. Hewitt, "Use of Statistical Analysis in Assessing Appropriate Documentation and Coding," *Topics in Health Information Management*, Vol. 21, No. 2, 2000, pp. 41–50.

Rutledge, Robert, David Hoyt, A. Brent Eastman, Michael J. Sise, Thomas Velky, Timothy Canty, Thomas Wachtel, and Turner M. Osler, "Comparison of the Injury Severity Score and ICD-9 Diagnosis Codes as Predictors of Outcome in Injury: Analysis of 44,032 Patients," *The Journal of Trauma: Injury, Infection, and Critical Care*, Vol. 42, No. 3, March 1997, pp. 477–489.

Rutledge, Robert, and Turner Osler, "The ICD-9 Based Illness Severity Score: A New Model That Outperforms Both DRG and APR-DRG as Predictors of Survival and Resource Utilization," *The Journal of Trauma: Injury, Infection, and Critical Care*, Vol. 45, No. 4, October 1998, pp. 791–799.

Schneider, Eric C., Virginia Riehl, Sonja Courte-Wienecke, David M. Eddy, and Cary Sennett, "Enhancing Performance Measurement: NCQA's Road Map for a Health Information Framework," *JAMA*, Vol. 282, No. 12, September 22/29, 1999, pp. 1184–1190.

Schulz, S., A. Zaiss, R. Brunner, D. Spinner, and R. Klar, "Conversion Problems Concerning Automated Mapping from ICD-10 to ICD-9," *Methods of Information in Medicine*, No. 37, 1998, pp. 254–259.

State of California, Office of Statewide Health Planning and Development, "Patient Discharge Data for California," www.oshpd.cahwnet.gov/HQAD/HIRC/patient/discharges/index.htm.

Taylor, C. Barr, et al., "Evaluation of a Nurse-Care Management System to Improve Outcomes in Patients with Complicated Diabetes," *Diabetes Care,* Vol. 26, 2003, pp. 1058–1063.

Tully, Lorraine, and Vera Rulon, "Evolution of the Uses of ICD-9-CM Coding: Medicare Risk Adjustment Methodology for Managed Care Plans," *Topics in Health Information Management*, Vol. 21, No. 2, 2000, pp. 62–67.

Turnbull, Gwen B., "The Truth About Medical Codes: It's More Than a Bunch of Numbers," *Ostomy/Wound Management,* Vol. 48, No. 11, November 2002, pp. 10–12.

Udris, Edmunds M., David Au, Mary B. McDonnell, Leway Chen, Donald C. Martin, William Tierney, and Stephan Fihn, "Comparing Methods to Identify General Internal Medicine Clinic Patients with Chronic Heart Failure," *American Heart Journal*, Vol. 142, No. 6, December 2001, pp. 1003–1009.

Williams, G. Rhys, John G. Jiang, David B. Matchar, and Gregory P. Samsa, "Incidence and Occurrence of Total (First-Ever and Recurrent) Stroke," *Stroke*, Vol. 30, No. 12, December 1999, pp. 2523–2528.

Workgroup for Electronic Data Interchange (WEDI), "Issues Surrounding the Proposed Implementation of ICD-10," http://www.wedi.org/cmsUploads/pdfUpload/eventsPresentationInformation/pub/icd-10wediwhitepaper3-24-2000.pdf.

Wysowski, Diane, Joslyn Swann, and Amarilys Vega, "Use of Isotretinoin (Accutane) in the United States: Rapid Increase from 1992 Through 2000," *Journal of the American Academy of Dermatology*, Vol. 46, No. 4, pp. 505–509.

TM91880-H